ECG Interpretation

pocket tutor

ECG
Interpretation

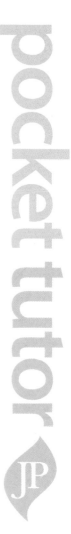

pocket tutor

Simon James MBBS MRCP
Consultant Electrophysiologist
James Cook University Hospital
Middlesbrough, UK

Katharine Nelson MBBS MRCP
Specialty Trainee in Cardiology
James Cook University Hospital
Middlesbrough, UK

JP
medical
publishers

© 2011 JP Medical Ltd.

Published by JP Medical Ltd, 83 Victoria Street, London, SW1H 0HW, UK

Reprinted 2014

Tel: +44 (0)20 3170 8910   Fax: +44 (0)20 3008 6180

Email: info@jpmedpub.com   Web: www.jpmedpub.com

ISBN: 978-1-907816-03-1

British Library Cataloguing in Publication Data
A catalogue record for this book is available from the British Library

Library of Congress Cataloging in Publication Data
A catalog record for this book is available from the Library of Congress

JP Medical Ltd is a subsidiary of Jaypee Brothers Medical Publishers (P) Ltd, New Delhi, India (www.jaypeebrothers.com).

Publisher:	Richard Furn
Development Editor:	Paul Mayhew
Copy Editor:	Julie Gorman
Design:	Pete Wilder, Designers Collective Ltd

Typeset, printed and bound in India.

Foreword

It is just over one hundred years since the very first recording that we would recognise as a modern electrocardiogram (ECG) was made by Willem Einthoven in 1903. This technique has since become one of the most useful clinical investigations available. There is an ECG machine on almost every hospital ward, in almost every doctor's office or practice, and in many emergency service vehicles. Almost every patient will at some time get an ECG, and since we are all likely to be patients at some stage in our life we shall all have our very own ECG recorded.

It is surprising, however, that very few of the doctors that record and use ECGs are really comfortable with interpreting the trace, and the majority rely on a machine-read analysis of the ECG or on a manual over-read by an expert colleague. Some ECG machine manufacturers have speculated that such is the general ignorance of the medical profession about how to read an ECG that the trace itself could be dispensed with and only the machine report might be produced. Those of us who do read ECGs, however, know that ECG machines often misdiagnose the trace, particularly when no clinical information or previous recordings are accessible to aid the diagnostic process. It therefore seems necessary that most of us who use the ECG should understand its normal configuration and the way it changes in the presence of disease.

There are already many ECG manuals, notebooks, primers and multivolume texts. Why is this new book a worthwhile contribution? The reason is that it is written by young and enthusiastic authors with a passion to educate and teach. Simon James and Katharine Nelson have written a small book that fits in the pocket and takes the reader from A to Z as far as the ECG is concerned.

It can be read from cover to cover or used as a reference when needed. It is illustrated beautifully and it is a real pleasure and education to read.

John Camm
British Heart Foundation Professor of Clinical Cardiology
St. George's University of London
London, United Kingdom

Preface

We're going to stick our necks out and declare that, history and examination aside, the 12-lead electrocardiogram (ECG) is the best diagnostic test available in modern medicine. This humble piece of A4 paper costs little, takes seconds to acquire, and presents no risk to the patient, yet it provides reliable, reproducible, internationally understood information concerning the human heart. From acute myocardial infarction to potentially fatal arrhythmias, the instant diagnosis made by ECG allows prompt delivery of life-saving treatment. A single 12-lead ECG can identify individuals at risk of ischaemic heart disease and stroke, two of the biggest killers in the western world. In the case of cardiac arrhythmias the ECG can identify those with potentially curable conditions as well as those at risk of sudden death, thereby allowing preventative measures to be taken.

In this book we attempt to teach the interpretation of ECGs from step one. A sound knowledge of the anatomy and physiology of the heart, together with a solid understanding of how the ECG is constructed, provides the clinician with the building blocks required for its interpretation up to the highest levels. These are provided in chapters 1–3. Theoretical understanding, however, is no substitute for seeing examples of 'real life' ECGs. For this reason, the main body of this book (chapters 4–12) is made up of clinical examples covering a broad range of important cardiac conditions. Each condition is described on a double page spread: short descriptive text and a labelled ECG facing each other on adjacent pages for ease of use.

We hope that you will enjoy reading this book and that the knowledge you gain will guide you in providing thoughtful, thorough and informed patient care.

Simon James
Katharine Nelson
May 2011

Contents

Acknowledgements

Thanks to the cardiology team at James Cook University Hospital for their help and support. Also to Paul Mayhew and Richard Furn at JP Medical Publishers for their indispensable guidance and patience. Thanks to Kerry, Lewis and Emily for looking after me and keeping me sane.

SJ

Thanks to all of my friends and colleagues for their help, advice and support. Also to JP Medical Publishers for their guidance and their patience throughout the writing and editorial process. Finally, my love and gratitude to Stuart, without whom very little would be possible.

KN

We gratefully acknowledge Prof ABM Abdullah whose book *ECG in Medical Practice, Third Edition*, published by Jaypee Brothers Medical Publishers (P) Ltd provided the source for 29 of the redrawn ECGs in this book.

SJ, KN

First principles

1.1 Anatomy

The heart is vital for human life. It is made of specialised muscle and is responsible for pumping blood to all the organs and tissues via the arteries.

Embryologically, the heart is derived from the mesodermic cell layer during the third week of gestation. This group of cells, called the mesocardium, differentiates to form the various layers of the heart: the endothelium, myocardium, epicardium and pericardium (**Figure 1.1**).

The heart is situated in the middle of the thorax, slightly off-set to the left. On examination the heart is felt and heard more strongly on the left due to the larger, stronger left ventricle.

Systemic and pulmonary circulations

The human heart consists of four chambers: two receiving chambers, the *atria*, and two pumping chambers, the *ventricles*

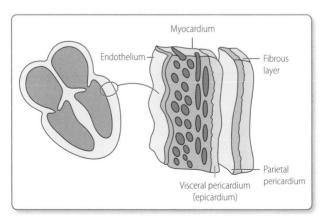

Figure 1.1 The layers of the heart.

(**Figure 1.2**). These form two separate circulatory routes, the *pulmonary circulation* delivering blood to and from the lungs, and the *systemic circulation* delivering blood to and from the rest of the body. The cardiac chambers are separated by valves, which ensure that there is no backflow of blood, and provide electrical insulation between the atria and the ventricles.

Deoxygenated blood from the body returns to the right atrium via the *superior and inferior venae cavae*. There is passive flow of blood from the right atrium into the right ventricle, followed by contraction of the right atrium to push more blood through the *tricuspid valve* into the right ventricle (**Figure 1.3**). The right ventricle then contracts, forcing the tricuspid valve to shut and ejecting blood though the *pulmonary valve* to the pulmonary arteries and on to the lungs. At the lung capillary

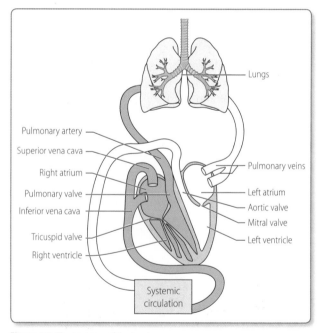

Figure 1.2 The anatomy of the heart.

1. Atrial systole

- Atria contract, ventricles relaxed
- Tricuspid and mitral valves open
- Blood forced into ventricles
- Pulmonary and aortic valves closed

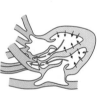

2. Early ventricular systole

- Atria relax, ventricles contract
- Tricuspid and mitral valves close
- Pulmonary and aortic valves still closed

3. Late ventricular systole

- Atria relax, ventricles contract
- Tricuspid and mitral valves closed
- Blood ejected from ventricles
- Pulmonary and aortic valves forced open

4. Early ventricular diastole

- Atria and ventricles relax
- All valves closed
- Atria begin filling with blood

5. Late ventricular diastole

- Atria and ventricles relax
- Tricuspid and mitral valves open
- Blood starts to enter ventricles
- Pulmonary and aortic valves closed

Figure 1.3 The cardiac cycle.

beds, gas exchange occurs and the blood becomes oxygenated. It then travels onwards via the *pulmonary veins* back to the heart, arriving at the left atrium.

At the left atrium there is passive flow of oxygenated blood into the left ventricle, followed by atrial contraction, which pushes more blood through the *mitral valve* into the left ventricle. The left ventricle is required to generate great pressure to deliver blood to the body, and consequently has greater muscle mass than the right ventricle. When the left ventricle contracts, the *mitral valve* closes and blood is propelled through the *aortic valve* into the *aorta*. From there oxygenated blood is distributed to the organs and tissues of the body, where oxygen delivery occurs at the capillary beds. The deoxygenated blood returns via the venous system to the *venae cavae*, and then to the right atrium.

Coronary circulation

The heart, like any other muscle, requires a blood supply in order to provide it with the necessary supplies required for metabolism and contraction. The heart receives its oxygenated blood via the coronary arteries (**Figure 1.4**).

These vessels arise from the aorta just beyond the aortic valve (**Figure 1.5**). In most people the right and left coronary

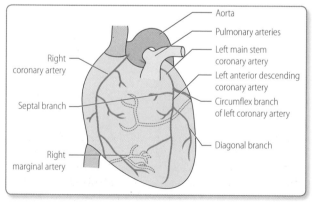

Figure 1.4 The heart and the coronary arteries.

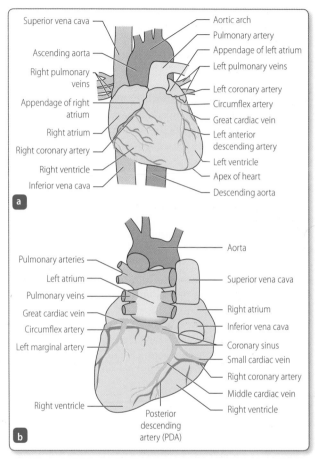

Figure 1.5 The superficial features of the heart.

arteries originate from the corresponding sides of the aorta. The right coronary artery supplies blood to the right ventricle and the inferior part of the left ventricle. It also gives branches to the right atrium, including the *sinoatrial (SA) node* and gives a branch to the *atrioventricular (AV) node*. The left main stem of the coronary artery divides into two large arteries. The left circumflex artery supplies the posterior part of the left ventricle. The left anterior descending artery supplies a large area of the left ventricle, including the anterior portion and apex, the septum (via septal branches) and the lateral aspect (via diagonal branches).

The anatomy of the conducting system

The left and right atria lie superiorly and are separated by the *interatrial septum* (**Figure 1.6**). The right atrium is derived from two embryological parts: the smooth walled venous (posterior) component is derived from the *sinus venosus*, and the muscular anterior part is derived from the rudimentary right atrium. Where the two fuse there is a vertical crest that extends from the superior to the inferior vena cava. This is known as the *crista terminalis*.

The *SA node* is located adjacent to the crista terminalis in the right atrium and lies inferior to the superior vena cava. This area of specialised cardiac cells forms the heart's own 'pacemaker'.

Where the superior part of the crista terminalis meets the interatrial septum it gives rise to a specialised conduction pathway that conducts to the left atrium. This is known as *Bachmann's bundle*.

The atria are connected to their corresponding ventricles via the atrioventricular valves: the *tricuspid valve* lies between the right atrium and the right ventricle, and the *mitral valve* lies between the left atrium and the left ventricle.

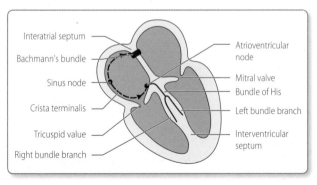

Figure 1.6 The anatomy of the conducting system.

The mitral and tricuspid valves and their associated annuli electrically insulate the ventricles from the atria. The only electrical connection between the atria and the ventricles is through the *atrioventricular node*

> ## Guiding principle
>
> From an electrical perspective, the heart is seen as having only two (rather than four) chambers, one atrial and one ventricular, which are electrically insulated from each other by non-conducting cartilage tissue.

(AV node), which lies in the low right atrial septum near the tricuspid valve.

The AV node has two separate electrical inputs. The *fast pathway* originates in the atrial septum and enters the node anteriorly. The *slow pathway* is a continuation of the lower margin of the crista terminalis and enters the node posteriorly.

The AV node communicates directly with a specialised narrow tract of conducting tissue called the *bundle of His*. This bundle is at first a single pathway that runs in the membranous interventricular septum, but it subsequently divides into the right and *left bundle branches*, which run to the apex of the heart.

The left bundle divides further into the *anterior and posterior fascicles*. From the bundle branches, conduction myofibres (*Purkinje fibres*) spread throughout the ventricular myofibres. The His–Purkinje network has specialised, rapid conducting properties as compared with general myocardial conduction.

1.2 Physiology

Cardiac action potential

The heart consists of specialised muscle cells called *myocytes*. Muscle cell contraction is associated with the electrical discharge of these cells, and is called *depolarisation*. These electrical discharges can be detected and recorded at the surface of the body.

Cardiac cells have a resting membrane potential of –96 mV (**Figure 1.7a**). This means that there is a net negative charge inside the cell, maintained by membrane protein channels that

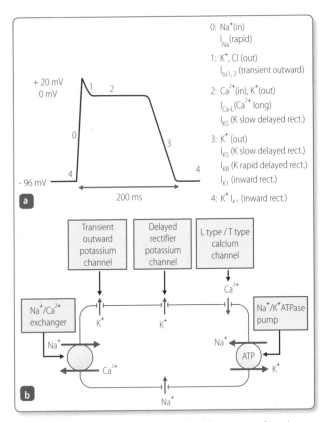

Figure 1.7 (a) the cardiac cell action potential and the sequence of membrane ion channel openings; (b) the movement of key cations (Na⁺, sodium; Ca²⁺, calcium, K⁺, potassium) in the cell.

control the movement of the key cations: sodium (Na^+): calcium (Ca^{2+}) and potassium (K^+) (**Figure 1.7b**). When the channels are stimulated by a neighbouring muscle cell (or by depolarisation of the SA node) they reach a certain threshold, triggering a chain of events. Rapid sodium channels open and sodium ions flow into the cell, resulting in rapid depolarisation. Next, slow calcium channels open inside the sarcolemma and sarcoplasmic reticulum, increasing the calcium level in the cytosol, and at the same time the cell membrane becomes less permeable to potassium, slowing the outflow of potassium ions. The overall effect is of balancing the membrane potential at around 0 mV for a prolonged 'plateau' phase. By this mechanism cardiac cells are able to depolarise and contract for longer. Finally, potassium channels reopen and calcium channels close, more potassium leaves the cell, less calcium enters and the negative membrane potential is restored – this is called *repolarisation*.

During the repolarisation period it is impossible to cause the cell to depolarise again. This is the refractory period.

Cardiac electrical network

During development of the heart a small number of heart muscle cells develop a property called *automaticity*, whereby they repeatedly and rhythmically depolarise, or 'fire' action potentials. The area of heart muscle with the highest rate of automaticity is the SA node, the heart's natural pacemaker, which usually initiates myocardial depolarisation.

The rate at which the SA node depolarises is influenced by parasympathetic stimulation via the vagus nerve (reduces the rate) and sympathetic stimulation (increases the rate) via the sympathetic nerves and circulating catecholamines. The result is a 'normal' resting heart rate of around 60–100 beats/min.

Guiding principle

Control of the sinoatrial node
- The SA node is the heart's natural pacemaker, as it spontaneously depolarises. The rate of depolarisation is controlled by two main mechanisms – neural (nerve) and hormonal influences.
- Neural control is via the vagus (Xth) nerve, which provides parasympathetic nervous input. During periods of rest or inactivity the input of this nerve reduces the rate of SA node depolarisation. Nerves from the T1–4 spinal level provide the sympathetic supply. During exercise or stress the input of these nerves increases the SA node rate and heart rate.
- Circulating hormones (particularly adrenaline and thyroxine) also affect SA node rate. Increasing levels of these hormones (e.g. due to exercise and thyroid disease, respectively) result in increased SA node rate and heart rate.

From the SA node the electrical impulse spreads to the right atrium through three intra-atrial pathways, while Bachmann's bundle carries the impulse to the left atrium.

Having activated the atria, the impulse enters the atrioventricular node; the brief delay that results allows time for the atrial contraction to finish, thus ensuring that sufficient blood is passed into the ventricles.

After the atrioventricular nodal delay, the impulse travels to the bundle of His, which then splits into the right bundle branch (RBB) (traversing the right ventricle) and a left bundle branch (LBB), which traverses the left ventricle and splits into the left posterior fascicle and a left anterior fascicle.

The *posterior fascicle* is a broad band of fibres that spreads over the posterior and inferior surfaces of the left ventricle. The *anterior fascicle* is a narrow band of fibres that spreads over the anterior and superior surfaces of the left ventricle.

Having traversed the bundle branches, the impulse finally passes into their terminal ramifications, the Purkinje fibres. These fibres traverse the thickness of the myocardium to activate the entire myocardial mass from the endocardial surface to the epicardial surface (i.e. inside to outside).

1.3   Cell physiology

Within the cardiac cells there are hundreds of *myofibrils*, which are long, thin structures made of thin and thick filaments. The thin filaments are composed of a protein called *actin*, and the thick filaments are made of a protein called *myosin*.

When the cardiomyocyte (**Figure 1.8**) is stimulated by an action potential it causes the sarcoplasmic reticulum to release calcium into the cell. This calcium allows myosin heads to bind to actin filaments and pull them together, causing the myofibrils to shorten. This is how electrical activity (the action potential) causes the individual muscle cells to contract. The action potential passes to adjacent cells directly via special channels called *gap junctions*, and in this way the contraction spreads throughout the heart.

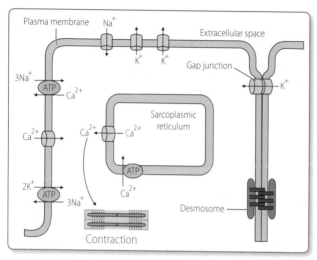

Figure 1.8 Cell physiology: the cardiomyocyte.

1.4 Electrical activity and the ECG

The electrical activity within the heart can be detected by electrodes placed on the skin. The record of the heart's electrical activity is known as the *electrocardiogram* (ECG).

The ECG is recorded using adhesive, disposable electrodes attached to different sites on the patient, and the trace is drawn onto paper with standard-sized squares.

The ECG machine is usually calibrated such that a 1 mV signal results in a deflection of 1 cm (two large squares) on the ECG recording. The calibration signal should be included with every recording. The recording paper speed is normally 25 mm/s. If no electrical signal is detected, a flat line will be drawn; this is called the *baseline*.

The direction of a deflection depends on two factors: the direction of spread of the electrical force and the location of the recording electrode. An electrical signal travelling towards an electrode is recorded as a positive deflection (above the

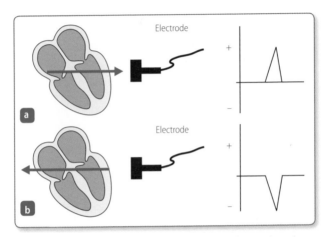

Figure 1.9 Electrical impulses travelling toward and away from an electrode result in positive and negative deflections, respectively.

baseline), and an electrical signal travelling away from an electrode is recorded as a negative deflection (below the baseline) (**Figure 1.9**).

Electrical activity is a vector quantity, i.e. it possesses both magnitude and direction. The size of a positive or negative deflection is determined by a combination of these two properties. For example, the ventricles have the greatest muscle mass, and therefore generate a larger electrical discharge (and consequently larger ECG complexes) than do the atria. However, the actual size of the complex recorded by the ECG will vary according to the location of electrode on the patient.

In the example shown in **Figure 1.10a**, the electrode is looking directly towards the direction of depolarisation. The vector component of electrical discharge towards the electrode is equal to its total magnitude and thus gives the maximum deflection on the ECG of 10 mV.

Guiding principle

The magnitude of the deflection seen on an ECG depends on the absolute size of the electrical discharge and its direction of propagation in relation to the electrode.

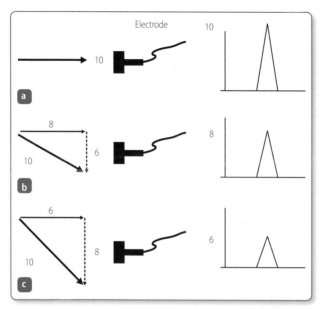

Figure 1.10 Vector summation according to the direction of depolarisation relative to the position of the electrode.

In **Figures 1.10b** and **1.10c** the electrode is located such that the depolarisation is travelling in an oblique direction towards it. As a vector quantity, the electrical discharge can be considered as being composed of two components at mutual right angles. For these oblique cases, the component of depolarisation heading directly towards the electrode is less, so that a weaker voltage is recorded. The more oblique the angle, the lower the voltage.

The importance of electrode location and the propagation vector is discussed further in Chapter 2.

The recorded ECG provides information about the electrical activity occurring at different times in the cardiac cycle. As multiple electrodes are used to record the ECG, the electrical activity at different cardiac sites can be assessed, with each lead providing a different 'window' onto a different part of the heart.

Understanding the normal ECG

2.1 Introduction

During activation of the myocardium, electrical forces (action potentials) are propagated in various directions. These electrical forces can be picked up from the surface of the body by means of electrodes and recorded in the form of an ECG.

A pair of electrodes, consisting of a positive and a negative electrode, constitutes an electrocardiographic *lead*. Each lead is oriented to record electrical forces as viewed from one particular aspect of the heart (**Figure 2.1**). By placing electrodes

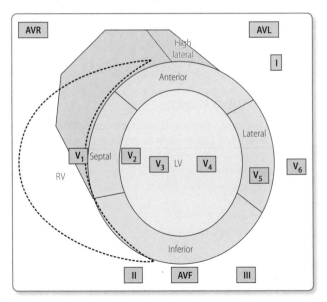

Figure 2.1 The 12-lead view of the heart. V_1–V_6, chest leads; LV, left ventricle; RV, right ventricle, I–III, standard limb leads. Augmented limb leads: aVF, augmented vector left foot; aVL, augmented vector left arm. Note: the twelfth lead aVR (augmented vector right arm) cannot be shown in this orientation.

in specific places on the body surface the heart can be viewed electrically from different angles.

It is important to understand that each lead can only record the sum total of electrical activity coming *towards* it at any given moment. Therefore, if all the electrical activity in the heart is spreading towards a lead, a large positive signal is recorded. If, however, *most* electrical activity is spreading towards a lead, but a smaller amount is moving away, a smaller positive signal will be recorded. Similarly, a less strong electrical signal (e.g. through a thinner part of heart muscle, or electrical signals not heading directly towards a lead but still detected by that lead) will result in a smaller positive recording on the ECG.

The ECG is therefore affected by variations not only in the shape and size of the heart, but also by where the electrodes are placed. There is an internationally recognised standard way to place electrodes, which gives 12 standard views of the heart: the 12-lead ECG (**Figure 2.2**). If done correctly, an ECG can be reliably interpreted, no matter where it was recorded.

The 12 ECG leads are:
- six limb leads or extremity leads
- six chest leads or precordial leads.

2.2 The limb leads

The limb leads are derived from electrodes placed on the limbs. An electrode is placed on each of the right arm, the left arm and the left leg. A further electrode on the right leg acts as a 'grounding' electrode (**Figure 2.3**). By looking at electrical signals travelling between different pairs of electrodes, we can derive six leads:
- three standard limb leads
- three augmented limb leads.

Standard (limb) leads

The standard (limb) leads record a graph of the electrical forces acting between two limbs at a time. Therefore, the standard leads are also called *bipolar leads*. In these leads, one limb carries a positive electrode and the other limb carries a negative electrode. There are three standard leads: I, II and III (**Figure 2.4**):

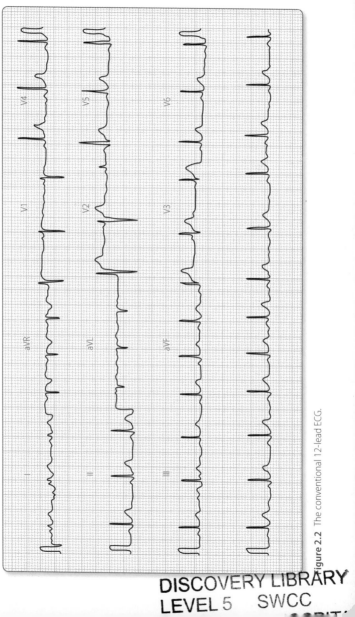

Figure 2.2 The conventional 12-lead ECG.

Lead	Positive electrode	Negative electrode
I	LA	RA
II	LL	RA
III	LL	LA

Where LA denotes left arm, LL left leg and RA right arm.

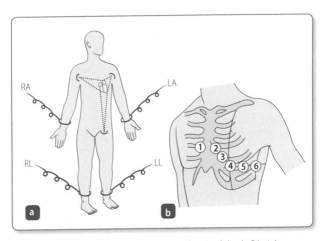

Figure 2.3 Electrode placement for ECG recording. Limb leads: RA, right arm; LA, left arm; RL, right leg; LL, left leg. Chest leads: V_1–V_6.

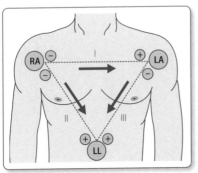

Figure 2.4 The three standard limb leads (bipolar leads) I–III. LA, left arm; LL, left leg; RA, right arm.

Augmented limb leads

The augmented limb leads give rise to a graph of the electrical forces as recorded from one limb at a time, and hence they are also known as *unipolar leads*. In these leads, one limb carries a positive electrode, while a central terminal provides the negative pole, which is measured as zero. There are three augmented limb leads (**Figure 2.5**):

Lead	Positive electrode
aVR	RA
aVL	LA
aVF	LL

- aVR (augmented vector right arm)
- aVL (augmented vector left arm)
- aVF (augmented vector left foot).

2.3 The chest leads

The chest leads are obtained from electrodes placed across the precordium. Electrodes are placed in six standard positions on the left side of the chest, each position representing one lead (see **Figure 2.1**)

- V_1: over the fourth intercostal space, just to the right of the sternum

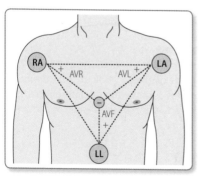

Figure 2.5 The three unipolar limb leads: aVR, aVL and aVF. LA, left arm; LL, left leg; RA, right arm.

- V_2: over the fourth intercostal space, just to the left of the sternum
- V_3: over a point midway between V_2 and V_4 (see V_4 below)
- V_4: over the fifth intercostal space in the midclavicular line
- V_5: over the anterior axillary line, at the same level as lead V_4
- V_6: over the midaxillary line, at the same level as leads V_4 and V_5.

Sometimes, the chest leads are configured with the electrodes placed on the right side of the chest. The right-sided chest leads are V_{1R}, V_{2R}, V_{3R}, V_{4R}, V_{5R} and V_{6R}, and these are mirror images of the standard left-sided chest leads:

- V_{1R}: over the fourth intercostal space, just to the left of the sternum
- V_{2R}: over the fourth intercostal space, just to the right of the sternum
- V_{3R}: over a point midway between V_{2R} and V_{4R}
- V_{4R}: over the fifth intercostal space in the midclavicular line
- V_{5R}: over the anterior axillary line, at the same level as lead V_{4R}
- V_6: over the midaxillary line, at the same level as leads V_{4R} and V_{5R}.

The right-sided chest leads are particularly useful for the assessment of the right ventricle.

2.4 The lead orientation

The 12-lead ECG consists of the following 12 leads recorded simultaneously:

I   II   III   aVR   aVL   aVF V_1 V_2 V_3 V_4 V_5 V_6

By considering the surface anatomy of the heart (**Figure 2.6**), we can see that most leads overlie or 'look at' the dominant, and more clinically important, left ventricle. Different parts of the left ventricle are viewed with different leads, as shown in **Table 2.1**.

The Einthoven triangle

We have seen that the standard limb leads are recorded from two limbs at a time, one carrying the positive electrode and the

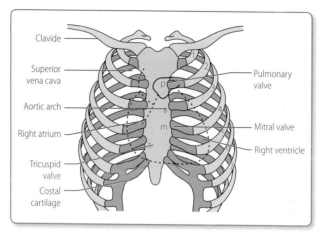

Figure 2.6 The surface anatomy of the heart.

ECG leads	Region of left ventricle
V_1, V_2	Septal
V_3, V_4	Anterior
V_5, V_6	Lateral
V_1 to V_4	Anteroseptal
V_3 to V_6	Anterolateral
I, aVL	High lateral
II, III, aVF	Inferior

Table 2.1 The region of the left ventricle represented on the ECG

other, the negative electrode. The three standard limb leads (I, II, III) can be seen to form an equilateral triangle, with the heart at the centre. This is called the *Einthoven triangle* (**Figure 2.7**).

To facilitate the graphical representation of electrical forces, the three limbs of the Einthoven triangle can be redrawn in such a way that the three leads they represent bisect each other and pass through a common central point. This produces a triaxial reference system with each axis separated from the next by 60°, the lead polarity (positive and negative poles) and orientation (direction) remaining the same (**Figure 2.7**).

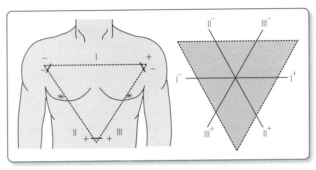

Figure 2.7 The Einthoven triangle of limb leads. The triaxial reference system.

We have also seen that the augmented limb leads are recorded from one limb at a time, the limb carrying the positive electrode and the negative pole being represented by the central point. The three augmented limb leads (aVR, aVL, aVF) form another triaxial reference system, with each axis being separated from the next by 60° (**Figure 2.8a**).

When this triaxial system of unipolar leads is superimposed on the triaxial system of limb leads, we can derive a hexaxial reference system with each axis being separated from the next by 30° (**Figure 2.8b**). Note that each of the six leads retains its polarity (positive and negative poles) and orientation (lead direction).

The hexaxial reference system is important in determining the major direction of the heart's electrical forces. As we shall

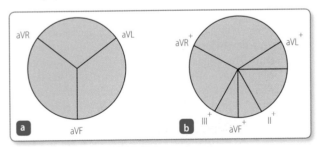

Figure 2.8 The triaxial reference system from unipolar leads. The hexaxial system from unipolar and limb leads.

see later, this is what is called the electrical axis of the QRS complex. Using this approach, specific points of pathology can be located, as the ECG is an abstract three-dimensional map of the heart's electrical activity.

2.5 ECG nomenclature

The ECG is composed of a series of deflections or waves. The distances between sequential waves on the time axis are called *intervals*. Portions of the isoelectric line (baseline) between successive waves are called *segments*.

For ECG and electrical purposes the heart is thought of as having two chambers: the biatrial chamber and the biventricular chamber (**Figure 2.9**). This is because the atria are activated together and then the ventricles contract synchronously. Therefore, on the ECG, atrial activation is represented by a single wave and ventricular activation by a single wave complex.

The wave of excitation is synchronised so that the atria and the ventricles contract and relax in a rhythmic sequence. Atrial depolarisation is followed by atrial repolarisation, which is nearly synchronous with ventricular depolarisation; finally, ventricular repolarisation occurs.

Cardiac contraction (systole) and relaxation (diastole) are mechanical events that are coupled with the heart's electrical

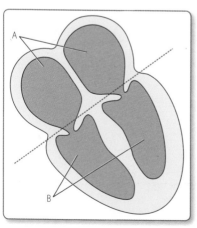

Figure 2.9 The dual-chamber concept: A, biatrial chamber; B, biventricular chamber.

behaviour. Depolarisation just precedes systole, and repolarisation is immediately followed by diastole.

ECG deflections

Each electrocardiographic deflection has been assigned a letter of the alphabet. Accordingly, a complete sequence of a single cardiac cycle is sequentially termed as P, Q, R, S, T and U (**Figure 2.10**). Each deflection represents different parts of the cardiac cycle:

- P wave: atrial depolarisation
- QRS complex: ventricular depolarisation
- Q wave: the first negative deflection before the R wave
- R wave: the first positive deflection after the Q wave
- S wave: the first negative deflection after the R wave
- T wave: ventricular repolarisation
- U wave: Purkinje system repolarisation (**Figure 2.11**).

Atrial repolarisation is not visualised on the ECG because it coincides with (and is therefore buried in) the larger QRS complex.

P, T and U waves are always denoted by capital letters. The Q, R and S waves are represented by either a capital letter or a small letter, depending on their relative or absolute magnitude. Large waves (over 5 mm) are assigned capital letters Q, R and S, while small waves (under 5 mm) are assigned lower case letters q, r and s.

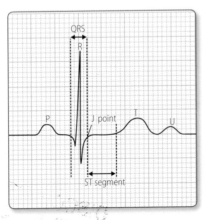

Figure 2.10 The normal ECG deflections.

Relatively speaking, a small q followed by a tall R is termed a qR complex, while a large Q followed by a small r is termed a Qr complex (**Figure 2.12**). Similarly, a small r followed by a deep S is termed an rS complex, while a large R followed by a small s is termed an Rs complex .

If a QRS deflection is totally negative without any positive deflection, it is termed a QS complex.

Furthermore, if the QRS complex reflects two positive waves, the second positive wave is denoted by R′ and the complex is termed rSR′ or RsR′ depending on magnitude of the positive (r or R) wave and the negative (s or S) wave.

Intervals and segments

The distances between certain ECG waves are relevant in order to establish a temporal relationship between events during a

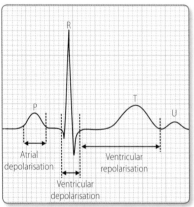

Figure 2.11 Depolarisation and repolarisation depicted as deflections.
Note: atrial repolarisation is buried in the QRS complex.

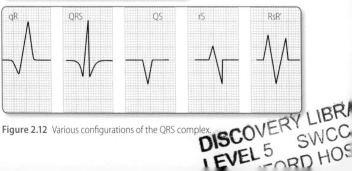

Figure 2.12 Various configurations of the QRS complex.

cardiac cycle. As the distance between waves is expressed on a time axis, these distances are termed *ECG intervals*. Portions of the isoelectric line (baseline) between successive waves are called *segments*. The ECG intervals and segments described below are clinically important.

PR interval

The PR interval is measured from the onset of the P wave to the beginning of the QRS complex, irrespective of whether the initial QRS deflection is positive or negative (**Figure 2.13**). The duration of the P wave is included in the measurement.

The PR interval is an estimate of atrioventricular conduction time. This includes the time for atrial depolarisation (P wave), conduction delay in the atrioventricular node and the time required for the impulse to transverse the ventricular conduction system before ventricular depolarisation (QRS) ensues.

PR segment

The PR segment is that portion of the isoelectric line that intervenes between the termination of the P wave and the onset of

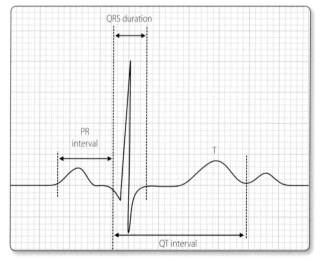

Figure 2.13 The normal ECG intervals.

the QRS complex (**Figure 2.14**). This segment does not include the width of the P wave. Inflammatory conditions can result in changes in the PR segment (e.g. pericarditis).

QT interval

The QT interval is measured from the onset of the Q wave to the end of the T wave (see **Figure 2.13**). If it is measured to the end of the U wave, it is termed the QU interval. The duration of the QRS complex, the length of the ST segment and the duration of the T wave are included in the measurement.

As the QRS complex represents ventricular depolarisation and the T wave represents ventricular repolarisation, the QT interval is an expression of the total duration of the ventricular systole.

Figure 2.15 shows an example of calculating the QT interval. Here:

- The QT interval is 14 small squares (one small square is 40 ms), i.e. 560 ms
- The RR interval is 10 large squares. i.e. 2 seconds (remember that the RR interval is measured in seconds)

$$QTc = \frac{QT}{\sqrt{RR}} = \frac{560}{\sqrt{2}} = \frac{560}{1.4} = 400 \text{ ms}$$

So in this example the QT interval is long, but when adjusted for very slow heart rate (this patient was in complete heart block with a ventricular rate of 30 bpm) it is normal at 400 ms.

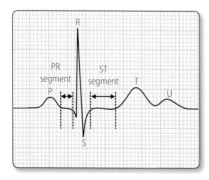

Figure 2.14 The normal ECG segments.

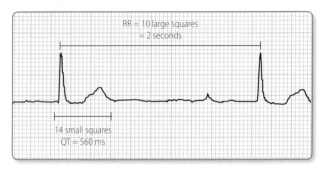

Figure 2.15 Calculating the QT interval

As the U wave represents Purkinje system repolarisation, the QU interval in addition takes into account the time taken for the ventricular Purkinje system to repolarise.

ST segment

The ST segment is that portion of the isoelectric line that intervenes between the termination of the S wave and the onset of the T wave (see **Figure 2.14**). The point at which the QRS complex ends and the ST segment begins is termed the junction point or J point (see **Figure 2.10**). The ST segment may be abnormal in many conditions, including ischaemic heart disease.

chapter 3

Interpreting the ECG: a six-step approach

Before interpreting the content of the ECG it is important to check that the basic details are correct:

- Is it the correct patient's name on the ECG for the patient in question?
- Is the ECG standardised? The paper speed should be 25 mm/s and the amplitude calibrated so that a 10 mm deflection represents 1 mV (**Figure 3.1**).

The actual interpretation of the ECG itself breaks down into three main areas:

- Rate
- Rhythm
- Specific pathological changes.

The first two components are most easily addressed using a six-step approach to examining the ECG:

1. Is there (ventricular) QRS electrical activity?
2. What is the rate of the QRS activity?
3. Is the QRS rhythm regular, regularly irregular or irregularly irregular?
4. Are the QRS complexes narrow (normal) or broad (> 120 ms)?
5. Is there atrial activity (e.g. P waves, fibrillation waves)?
6. How is the atrial activity (P wave) related to ventricular activity (QRS)?

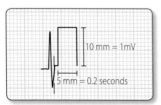

Figure 3.1 A standardising wave for an ECG.

10 mm = 1mV

5 mm = 0.2 seconds

These steps will iden-
tify the underlying cardiac
rhythm. Further analysis
of individual components
of the ECG helps to iden-
tify underlying pathological
changes, including struc-
tural abnormalities (e.g. old
infarction, hypertrophy),

Guiding principle

Cardiac rhythm

The cardiac rhythm is determined from the
lead that shows the P wave most clearly
(usually lead II). However, a single lead may
be recorded just to show the rhythm – this
is called a *rhythm strip*.

cardiac ischaemia, electrolyte imbalances or hereditary problems (e.g. long QT syndrome, Brugada syndrome).

Each of the above steps is now considered in turn.

3.1 Step 1: is there electrical activity?

The absence of any activity raises two possibilities. The patient
may be in *asystole* (a complete absence of any cardiac electrical
or mechanical activity); this would result in cardiac arrest
and is incompatible with life. The second possibility, and the
most likely in the awake/stable patient, is that the ECG is not
connected or recording accurately (most often a lead has
become disconnected).

3.2 Step 2: what is the QRS (ventricular) rate?

The normal ventricular rate is 60–100 beats/min. Rates slower
than 60 beats/min are called
bradycardic, and rates faster than 100 beats/min are
called *tachycardic*.

The rate can be calcu-
lated in two ways:

Guiding principle

- Tachycardia rate > 100 bpm (from the
  Greek: *tachy* = fast, *cardia* = heart)

- Bradycardia rate < 60 bpm (from the
  Greek: *brady* = slow, *cardia* = heart)

Method 1

Measure the distance (as the number of small squares) between
two successive ECG complexes. The number of ECG complexes
in 1 minute is equal to 1500 divided by that distance. This will
give the heart rate in beats per minute.

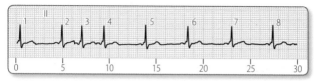

Figure 3.2 Step 2: example for Method 2.

Alternatively measure the distance between two successive complexes in large (5 mm) squares. Divide 300 by this number of squares to derive the rate in beats per minute.

Example:
1500 divided by 15 small squares = 100 beats/min
300 divided by 3 large squares = 100 beats/min

Method 2
If the rate varies from beat to beat, a better way to calculate the rate is by taking an average.

The ECG paper moves by 5 large squares (25 small squares) each second. Therefore, 30 large squares is equivalent to 6 seconds. Counting the number of complexes in this period and multiplying by 10 gives the approximate rate in beats per minute.
Example: sinus rhythm with ectopics at a rate of 8 beats in 30 large squares **(Figure 3.2)**
- There are 8 QRS complexes in a 6-second interval (30 large squares).
- Therefore the heart rate is around 8 × 10 = 80 beats/min.
   Some rate examples and traces are given in **Figure 3.3**.

3.3   Step 3: is the rhythm regular?

Is the interval between successive R waves or QRS complexes completely regular?

In **Figure 3.4a** the RR interval is regular, being unchanged for every pair of complexes. In **Figure 3.4b** the rate is now 150 beats/min (atrial flutter is the underlying rhythm) but the RR interval is still constant and the rhythm is *regular*.

In **Figure 3.4c** (sinus rhythm with bigeminy) the rhythm is irregular but in a predictable (regular) manner (alternating short and long RR intervals). Similarly, in **Figure 3.4d** (sinus rhythm with Mobitz type 2 block) the rhythm is irregular but with a

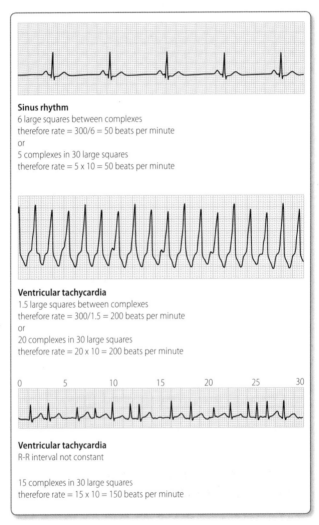

Sinus rhythm
6 large squares between complexes
therefore rate = 300/6 = 50 beats per minute
or
5 complexes in 30 large squares
therefore rate = 5 x 10 = 50 beats per minute

Ventricular tachycardia
1.5 large squares between complexes
therefore rate = 300/1.5 = 200 beats per minute
or
20 complexes in 30 large squares
therefore rate = 20 x 10 = 200 beats per minute

Ventricular tachycardia
R-R interval not constant

15 complexes in 30 large squares
therefore rate = 15 x 10 = 150 beats per minute

Figure 3.3 Step 2: examples of rates and the associated traces.

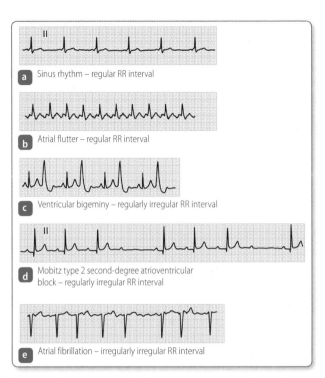

a Sinus rhythm – regular RR interval

b Atrial flutter – regular RR interval

c Ventricular bigeminy – regularly irregular RR interval

d Mobitz type 2 second-degree atrioventricular block – regularly irregular RR interval

e Atrial fibrillation – irregularly irregular RR interval

Figure 3.4 Step 3: variation in the RR interval: (a, b) regular; (c, d) regularly irregular; (e) irregularly irregular.

predictable pattern of three short RR intervals followed by a longer interval. The pattern then repeats. These two rhythms would be described as *regularly irregular*.

In **Figure 3.4e** (atrial fibrillation) the RR interval varies from beat to beat, with no predictable pattern. This rhythm is described as *irregularly irregular*.

3.4 Step 4: is the QRS narrow (normal) or broad?

A narrow (normal) QRS complex means that the ventricle must depolarise rapidly via a normal conducting system of the atrioventricular (AV) node–His bundle–bundle branches. This also means that the rhythm must originate from above the ventricles. For example, in sinus rhythm (**Figure 3.5a**), the rhythm propagates from the sinoatrial node across the atria to the AV node; the ventricles are depolarised via the His–Purkinje system. In SVT (**Figure 3.5b**) there is endless re-entry around the atria; the ventricles are depolarised via the AV node and then the His–Purkinje system. A narrow QRS complex is also seen in atrial arrhythmias.

A broad QRS (duration > 120 ms) suggests abnormal activation and delayed depolarisation of parts of the ventricle muscle. There are three possible explanations for this:

- The rhythm originates from a site within the ventricle but thereafter spreads in an eccentric way, i.e. other than via the His–Purkinje system system. Examples of this type are ventricular tachycardia (**Figure 3.5c**) and complete heart block (**Figure 3.5d**).
- The rhythm arises from above the ventricles but there is a problem within the conducting system that results in delayed activation of part of the ventricles. The most common example of this type is a block of either the left or the right bundle branch (**Figure 3.5e,f**).
- The rhythm arises from above the ventricle, but the ventricle is also activated by an extra pathway from the atrium. This results in part of the ventricle being activated earlier, and consequently in eccentric depolarisation of parts of the ventricle. An example of this type is Wolff–Parkinson–White syndrome (**Figure 3.5g**).

3.5   Step 5: is there atrial electrical activity?

In between the QRS complexes there may be electrical activity due to atrial depolarisations. These are most commonly P waves due to the spread of organised activity throughout the atria (see Chapter 2). However, there may be P waves present that have an unusual shape or rate (e.g. atrial tachycardia). Other possibilities include the chaotic irregular deflections of

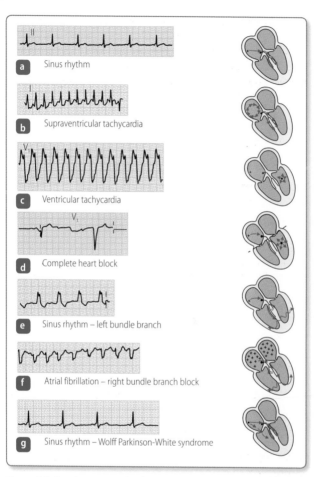

a Sinus rhythm

b Supraventricular tachycardia

c Ventricular tachycardia

d Complete heart block

e Sinus rhythm – left bundle branch

f Atrial fibrillation – right bundle branch block

g Sinus rhythm – Wolff Parkinson-White syndrome

Figure 3.5 Step 4: variation in the QRS complex. (a, b) Narrow (normal) QRS complex. (c–g) broad (abnormal) QRS complex due to a slower, eccentric pattern of depolarisation of the ventricle: (c, d) the rhythm originates from a site within the ventricle but thereafter spreads in a way other than via the His–Purkinje system; (e, f) the rhythm arises from above the ventricles but a problem within the conducting system results in delayed activation of part of the ventricles; (f) partial activation of the ventricle by the normal His–Purkinje network and partial activation via an accessory pathway.

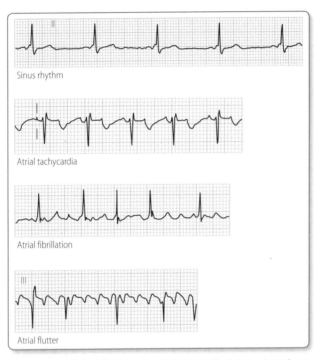

Sinus rhythm

Atrial tachycardia

Atrial fibrillation

Atrial flutter

Figure 3.6 Step 5: sinus rhythm, atrial tachycardia, atrial fibrillation and atrial flutter.

atrial fibrillation or the 'saw tooth' pattern seen in atrial flutter (**Figure 3.6**). In some instances there may be no visible atrial activity at all.

3.6 Step 6: how are atrial and ventricular activity related?

If atrial activity is present on the ECG, the next question is how does it relate to the ventricular activity? Is there one P wave for every QRS complex, or more (**Figure 3.7a**)? If there is a one-to-one relation, is the PR interval normal, short or long (**Figure 3.7b**)? Is the PR interval consistent or does it vary in pattern (Wenckebach; **Figure 3.7c**)? Alternatively, are the P waves completely unrelated to the QRS complexes

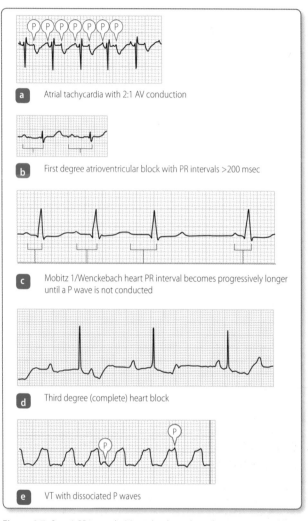

Figure 3.7 Step 6: PR intervals: (a) atrial tachycardia with a 2:1 response; (b) first-degree atrioventricular block, long PR interval; (c) second-degree heart block, Wenckebach phenomenon, progressive lengthening of the PR interval; (d) third-degree (complete) atrioventricular block, inconsistent PR intervals; (e) VT with dissociated P waves.

(complete AV block (**Figure 3.7d**); VT with dissociated P waves (**Figure 3.7e**)?

By following the above steps, the rate and rhythm can be easily and accurate assessed.

The next step is to assess the electrical axis – is it normal or does it deviate to the left or right (see Section 2.3)?

There is no specific system for confirming or excluding other specific pathological changes. It is more a case of looking in turn for the features of each condition that could be present. Examples include:

- slurred QRS onset/delta wave – Wolff–Parkinson–White syndrome
- large QRS voltages – left ventricular hypertrophy
- ST depression – myocardial ischaemia
- ST elevation – acute myocardial infarction.

> **Guiding principle**
>
> To make the systematic reading of ECGs second nature, practice applying it to any ECGs you come across in medical notes.

3.7 Glossary of distinct ECG signs

P mitrale   An abnormally notched and wide P wave, and usually most prominent in lead II; it is commonly seen in association with mitral valve disease, particularly mitral ste-

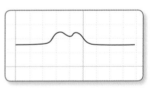

nosis. The diseased/narrowed mitral valve increases resistance to emptying and contraction of the left atrium, which is seen as the 'late' second bump of the elongated P wave.

P pulmonale   A peaked P wave amplitude in leads II, III and/or aVF is > 2.5 mm, it occurs due to right heart strain and is seen in pulmonary disease (e.g. chronic obstructive pulmonary disease, asthma, pul-

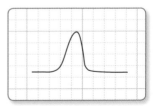

monary embolism) and chronic heart failure. The right atrium is overloaded against higher pressure in the right circulation, usually due to pulmonary disease, 'stretching' the atrial cardiomyocytes.

Long PR interval   Any PR interval as measured from the beginning of the P wave to the beginning of the QRS that is > 200 ms. This represents 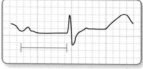 delayed conduction from the atria to the ventricles, most commonly due to age-related degeneration of the AV node.

Short PR interval   A PR interval < 80 ms. It may be normal or may represent the existence of an accessory pathway from the atria to the ventricles.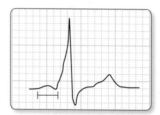

Delta wave   An upsloping segment of the PR segment, representing abnormal early conduction from the atria to the ventricles through an accessory pathway.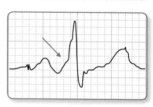

Broad QRS   QRS duration of > 120 ms, representing a slight delay between activation of the left and right ventricles. It may occur in a specific pattern, such as right or left bundle branch block.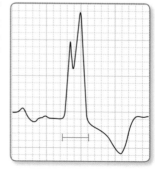

ST elevation   The normal ST segment is isoelectric (i.e. it is flat along the baseline). ST elevation may be a sign of acute myocardial infarction.

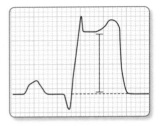

ST depression   Depression of the ST segment beneath the baseline. There are many causes, including cardiac ischaemia, left ventricular hypertrophy and digoxin use.

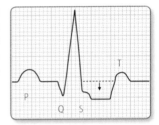

Long QT interval   A QT interval (corrected for the heart rate) of > 450 ms in men and 470 ms in women. It may be congenital or acquired.

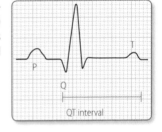

T wave inversion   A T wave that falls below the baseline, representing abnormal cardiac repolarisation. There are many causes, including cardiac ischaemia.

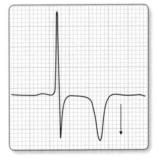

Flutter waves   A 'saw-tooth' baseline, representing a re-entry circuit somewhere in the atria.

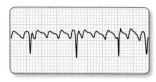

Fibrillation waves   An irregular baseline with no visible P waves, representing disordered atrial activity.

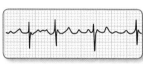

Ectopic beat   Cardiac depolarisation occurring outwith the normal expected cardiac cycle. It may be atrial, ventricular or junctional.

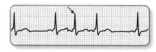

Bradyarrhythmias I: sinoatrial node dysfunction

A bradyarrhythmia is a disturbance in the heart rhythm where the heart rate is abnormally slow (usually under 60 beats/min). The bradyarrhythmias occur either due to failure of rhythm generation, or to failure of rhythm conduction. Failure of rhythm generation is usually due to the sinoatrial (SA) node not 'firing' at the normal rate. The SA node may fire continuously at a slower rate, resulting in ongoing bradycardia. Alternatively, it may have periods of firing at normal rates and periods of firing at slow rates, resulting in intermittent pauses.

Abnormal SA node function often causes symptoms but does not put the patient at risk of sudden death. The key to assessing these patients lies in their haemodynamic response to bradyarrhythmia. It should be ascertained whether the patient has a history of any syncope or presyncope, and the blood pressure, peripheral perfusion and level of consciousness should be checked. This information, together with the electrical diagnosis, will help in determining what kind of treatment is required and how quickly it must be given.

4.1 Sinus bradycardia (Figure 4.1)

Key features

- Heart rate is 60 beats/min
- A P wave before every QRS complex ①
- PR interval is normal (120–200 ms) ②
  The rate is calculated as shown.

Pathophysiology

The SA node depolarises consistently, but slower than normal. This may be due to disease (e.g. trauma or ischaemia) of the SA node itself, or to extrinsic causes influencing the rate of SA node depolarisation.

Clinical relevance

Sinus bradycardia is a normal finding in athletes, and in normal individuals when asleep. Pathological causes include SA node disease, drugs, increased vagal tone, hypothyroidism, uraemia, raised intracranial pressure and glaucoma.

Management

In normal individuals who are asymptomatic no treatment is needed. However, if the bradycardia is causing lightheadedness or blackouts, a cause should be sought and, if possible, reversed.

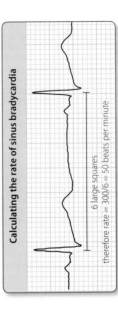

6 large squares

therefore rate = 300/6 = 50 beats per minute

Calculating the rate of sinus bradycardia

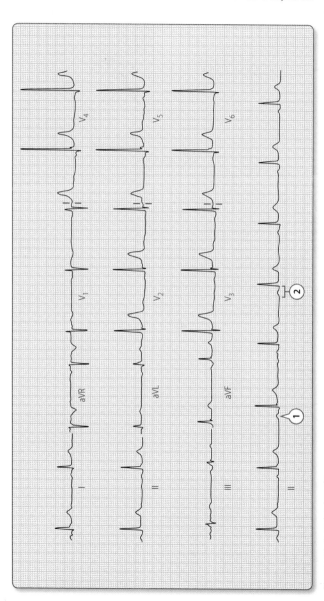

Figure 4.1 Sinus bradycardia.

4.2   Sinus pause with junctional escape beat (Figure 4.2)

Key features

- Abnormally long interval between one sinus beat and the next ①
- During the prolonged interval between sinus beats, other areas may depolarise as an 'escape rhythm'
- In the case shown here, a beat arising from near the AV node (junctional escape beat) occurs prior to the delayed next sinus beat (see junctional ectopic beat, Section 6.3) ②

Pathophysiology

The SA node fails to depolarise at the expected preceding rate. Due to its own 'automaticity' the AV node or 'junction' will depolarise, in order to avoid asystole.

Clinical relevance

Sinus pauses, with or without junctional escape beats, are not uncommon and are indeed a normal finding in many individuals, especially nocturnally. As a general rule, pauses are considered pathological if they last for longer than 3 s during waking hours, or if they are associated with symptoms.

Management

In normal individuals who are asymptomatic no treatment is needed. If symptoms do occur a cause should be sought, including electrolyte disturbances and medications that cause bradycardia. If no precipitating cause is found, or if there is one that cannot be reversed, a pacemaker may be implanted.

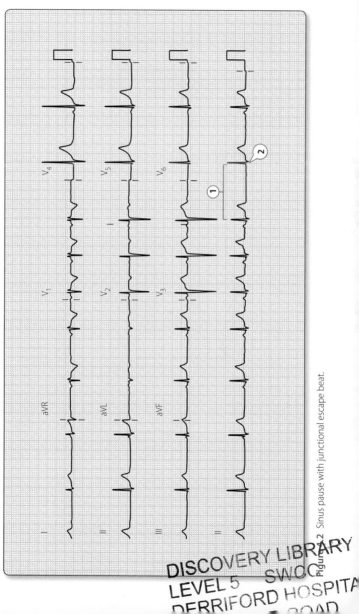

Figure 2 Sinus pause with junctional escape beat.

Bradyarrhythmias II: conduction abnormalities

Failure of conduction is the commonest cause of bradycardia. The most common reason for conduction failure is age-related fibrosis of the conduction system, which may be exacerbated or unmasked by rate-slowing cardiac drugs. The conducting system may be affected by myocardial infarction, or directly damaged through surgery or other cardiological procedures. Electrolyte imbalance, again potentially caused by drugs, is another common cause of bradyarrhythmias. Some conduction abnormalities merely indicate early disease of the conducting system (e.g. bundle branch block and first-degree heart block), while other abnormalities indicate advanced conduction disease (second- and third-degree heart block). These conditions are often symptomatic and may indicate that the patient is at risk of sudden death.

As for any bradycardia, assessing the patient's clinical status is vital. This will determine what kind of treatment is required and how quickly it must be undertaken. Warning signs include loss of consciousness, heart failure, chest pain and hypotension.

5.1   First-degree atrioventricular block (Figure 5.1)

Key features

- PR interval > 200 ms (5 small squares) ①
- Every P wave is followed by a QRS complex ②

Pathophysiology

P waves are consistently generated by the sinoatrial (SA) node, and these are consistently conducted down the His–Purkinje system. However, this process takes longer than in normal individuals, usually due to pathology affecting the atrioventricular (AV) node or an area high in the His bundle.

Clinical relevance

First-degree AV block is usually caused by age-related degeneration of the AV node or His bundle. It can, however, be a marker of progression of another disease (e.g. aortic root abscess in infective endocarditis, or calcific aortic stenosis). Drugs that suppress the AV node, such as calcium channel blockers, can also commonly cause first-degree AV block.

Management

Most individuals with first-degree AV block do not need any specific treatment. However, they should be assessed for secondary causes, and to review medications. If symptoms of bradyarrhythmia occur the patient should be monitored to ensure there is no higher degree AV block (second- or third-degree heart block).

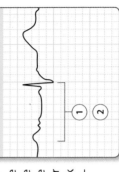

First-degree AV block: elongated PR interval

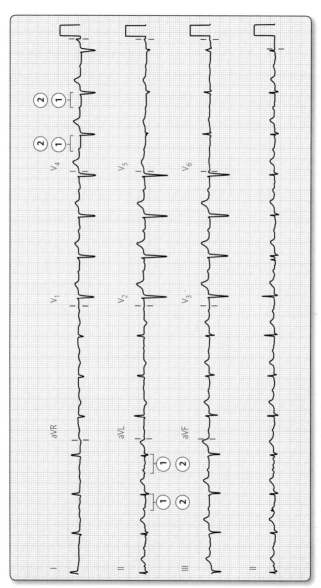

Figure 5.1 First-degree atrioventricular block.

5.2 Second-degree atrioventricular block: Mobitz type 1 or Wenckebach (Figure 5.2)

Key features

- PR interval becomes progressively longer with each beat, until eventually a P wave is not conducted; the process then begins again ①
- The pause that follows the non-conducted P wave is shorter than two normal sinus intervals

Pathophysiology

The SA node depolarises regularly in the usual fashion. Conduction through the AV node is impaired and becomes slower with each consecutive beat. Eventually a P wave reaches the AV node when it is still refractory (i.e. it is unable to conduct), and there is no QRS complex following that P wave.

Clinical relevance

Mobitz type 1 is a normal finding in healthy individuals, particularly in athletes or when it occurs at night. It can, however, represent underlying pathology, such as inferior myocardial infarction or toxicity (e.g. digoxin, beta blockers and calcium channel blockers).

Management

Asymptomatic individuals showing the Wenckebach phenomenon with no long pauses do not require any specific treatment. In those with symptoms, rate slowing drugs should be stopped where present. If symptoms persist a pacemaker is required.

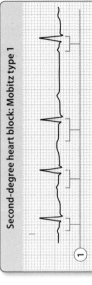

Second-degree heart block: Mobitz type 1

①

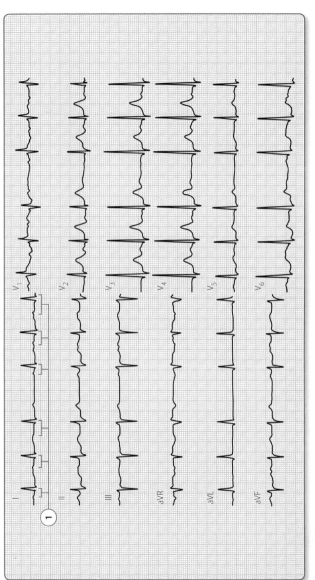

Figure 5.2 Second-degree atrioventricular block: Mobitz type 1 or Wenckebach.

5.3   Second-degree atrioventricular block: Mobitz type 2 (Figure 5.3)

Key features

- PR interval remains constant for conducted P waves ①
- P wave activity is regular, but not every P wave is followed by a QRS complex ②
- The next P wave conducts with the same PR interval as previously ③

Pathophysiology

The SA node depolarises normally. Degeneration of the conducting system below the AV node results in the tissue not recovering (repolarising) in time to conduct some impulses. Most P waves are conducted with a constant PR interval. Occasional P waves are not conducted to the ventricle.

The cause of Mobitz type 2 block include age-related degeneration, ischaemia or local infiltration (e.g. from aortic valve calcification).

Clinical relevance

Mobitz type 2 heart block is never a normal finding. It indicates significant disease in the conducting system of the heart, and carries a risk of asystole. Patients may present with fatigue, dizzy spells or syncope, or may be asymptomatic. All require early investigation and management.

Management

In the absence of a readily reversible cause patients in this heart rhythm require a permanent pacemaker, both to alleviate symptoms and to abolish the risk of asystole.

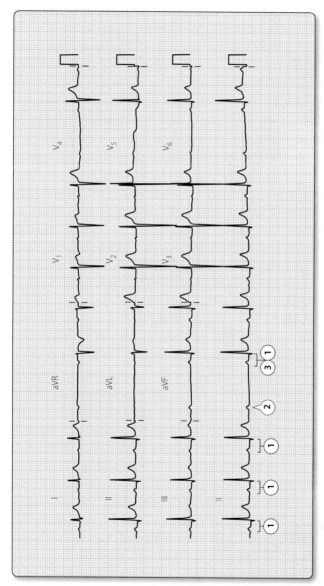

Figure 5.3 Second-degree atrioventricular block: Mobitz type 2.

5.4 Second-degree heart block: 2:1 atrioventricular block (Figure 5.4)

Key features

- P wave activity is regular, but not every P wave is followed by a QRS complex ①

- Every second P wave is not conducted – this is referred to as 2:1 conduction ②

- If every third P wave is followed by a QRS complex, this is referred to as 3:1 conduction.

Pathophysiology

The presence of 2:1 AV block implies degeneration of the conducting system below the level of the AV node. The distal conducting system fails to recover (repolarise) in time to conduct every second impulse to the ventricles. This can be caused by age-related degeneration, ischaemia or local infiltration (e.g. from aortic valve calcification). It may be aggravated by drugs that affect conduction, such as beta blockers and calcium channel blockers.

Clinical relevance

2:1 heart block indicates significant disease in the conducting system of the heart and carries a risk of asystole. Patients may present with fatigue, dizzy spells or syncope, or may be asymptomatic. All require early investigation and management.

Management

In the absence of a reversible cause, patients with this heart rhythm require a permanent pacemaker, both to alleviate symptoms and to minimise the risk of asystole.

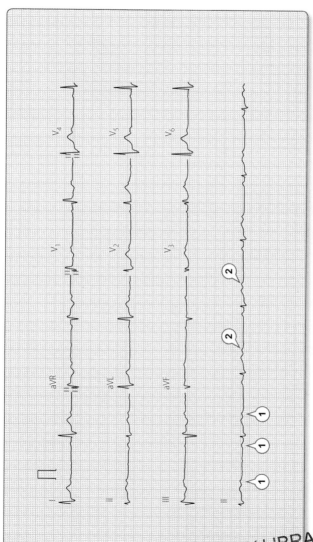

Figure 57 Second-degree 2:1 block.

5.5   Third-degree (complete) atrioventricular block: narrow QRS (Figure 5.5)

Key features

- Regular QRS with slow rate ①
- Complete dissociation of atrial and ventricular activity ②
- Varying PR interval ③
- Different atrial (P) and ventricular (QRS) rates
- Narrow QRS due to escape rhythm arising from AV node/junctional tissue ④

Pathophysiology

Loss of conduction results in no electrical communication between the atria and the ventricles. The ventricle relies on an escape rhythm arising just below the AV node or from the proximal His bundle (A). The rate is often faster than for broad QRS escape rhythms, and tends to be more reliable.

The atria and ventricles depolarise at independent rates, resulting in varying PR intervals, but constant PP intervals. Depolarisation spreads via the His–Purkinje system (B), and therefore the QRS complex is narrow.

Clinical relevance

Patients are often symptomatic due to bradycardia, and are at risk of asystole or cardiac arrest.

Management

A pacemaker is the treatment of choice, except in the rare cases with a reversible cause.

Sympathomimetics (adrenaline, isoprenaline, atropine) may be tried to increase the heart rate as a temporising measure prior to pacemaker implant.

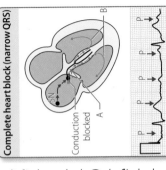

Complete heart block (narrow QRS)

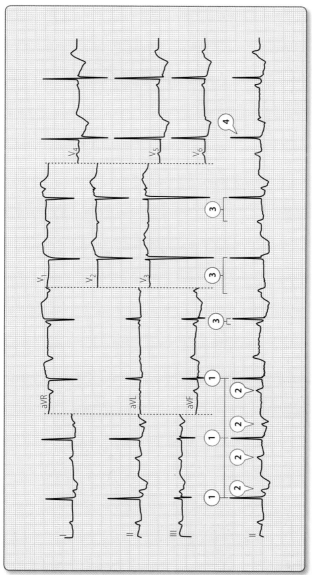

Figure 5.5 Third-degree (complete) atrioventricular block: narrow QRS.

5.6 Third-degree (complete) atrioventricular block: broad QRS (Figure 5.6)

Key features

- Regular QRS with slow rate ①
- Complete dissociation of atrial and ventricular activity ②
- Varying PR interval ③
- Different atrial and ventricular rates ④
- Broad QRS due to ventricular escape rhythm ⑤

Pathophysiology

Loss of conduction either through the AV node or the distal conducting tissue results in no electrical communication between the atria and ventricles. The ventricle relies on an escape rhythm of its own, which is usually 40 beats/min or slower.

The atria and ventricles depolarise at independent rates. Depolarisation is eccentric and not via the His–Purkinje system; slow propagation manifests as a broad QRS.

Clinical relevance

Patients are often symptomatic due to bradycardia, presenting with breathlessness, lethargy or syncope. They are at risk of asystole or cardiac arrest.

Management

See 5.5 Management (page 58).

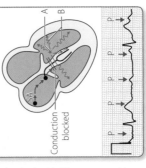

Complete heart block (broad QRS)

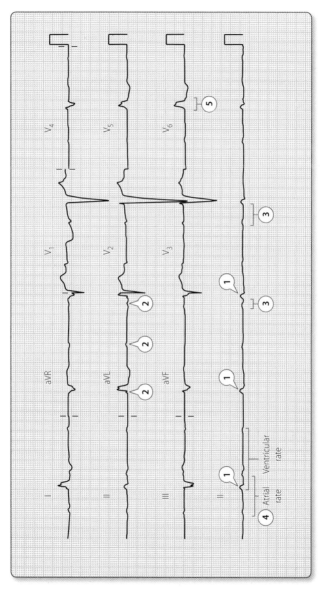

Figure 5.6 Third-degree (complete) atrioventricular block: broad QRS.

5.7 Right bundle branch block (Figure 5.7)

Key features

- Broad QRS complexes (> 120 ms or 3 small squares) ①
- There is a second positive deflection in the QRS complex – an rSR' pattern ②
- Slurring of the S wave laterally (leads V_5, V_6, I and aVL) ③
- T wave inversion in the septal leads ④

Pathophysiology

The right bundle branch of the His–Purkinje system does not conduct. All electrical signals travel down the left bundle branch. The septum is activated left to right (towards V_1) (**A**); the left ventricle depolarises (away from V_1) (**B**); depolarisation of the right ventricle (towards V_1) is delayed (**C**).

Right bundle branch block (RBBB) may be a normal finding or may be caused by, for example:

- fibrotic degeneration
- ischaemic heart disease
- congenital heart disease
- hypertension
- pulmonary embolus.

Clinical relevance

Consider the clinical context when investigating underlying cause. Further investigation may be needed (e.g. echocardiogram).

Management

RBBB in itself requires no specific treatment.

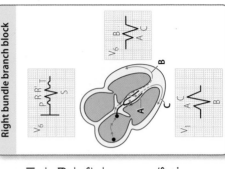

Right bundle branch block

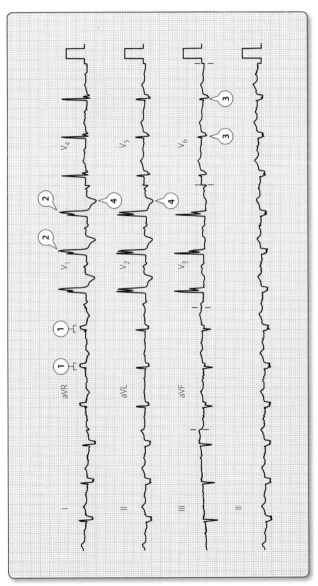

Figure 5.7 Right bundle branch block.

5.8 Left bundle branch block (Figure 5.8)

Key features

- Broad QRS (duration > 120 ms or 3 little squares) ①
- Abnormal morphology of QRS: W-shaped in V_1 and M-shaped in V_6 ②
- QRS onset is sharp or normal ③
- No R wave in leads V_1–V_4 ④
- ST elevation in the anterior leads, with T wave inversion laterally
- Underlying rhythm is sinus rhythm

Pathophysiology

Left bundle branch block (LBBB) represents delayed or absent conduction in either the left main bundle before it splits, or in both of the fascicles of the His–Purkinje system. As a result, the septum is activated in right to left direction (**A**) – away from V_1. Shortly afterwards the right ventricle depolarises as normal towards V_1 (**B**). The left ventricle depolarises late – away from V_1 (**C**).

This pattern of activation results in a W-shaped QRS complex in V_1 and a reciprocal M-shaped QRS in V_6. ST abnormalities are due to the altered pattern of repolarisation.

Causes of LBBB include:

- hypertension
- fibrotic degeneration
- ischaemic heart disease
- aortic stenosis
- cardiomyopathy.

Clinical relevance

LBBB is rarely a normal finding. It usually represents conduction disease due to scarring.

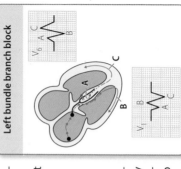

Left bundle branch block

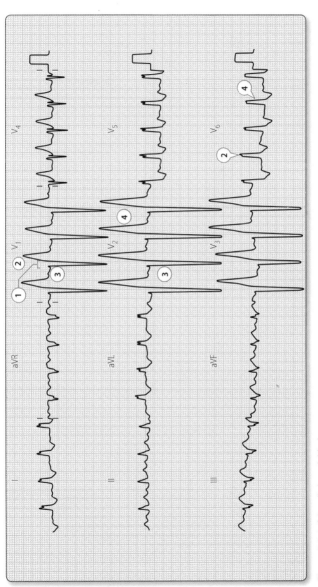

Figure 5.8 Left bundle branch block.

LBBB makes further interpretation of the ECG difficult. Rhythm problems are usually readily identifiable but supraventricular tachycardias will have a broad QRS complex, and thus they are sometimes confused with ventricular tachycardia. The ST segment and T wave will not show the usual changes associated with ischaemia, although serial ECGs recorded in and out of pain may show changes.

Acute myocardial infarction can present with new LBBB. In the absence of previous ECGs it can be very difficult to decide whether or not LBBB represents a new heart attack.

Management

There is no specific treatment for LBBB. Management is targeted to establishing and treating the underlying cause.

Ectopic beats

The term 'ectopic' means 'in the wrong place'. Thus, with regard to the ECG, ectopic beats are cardiac signals generated from anywhere other than the SA node. Essentially any part of the heart may act as a source of ectopic beats, but common sites include the atria, the AV node, the AV junction, and the ventricles. Beats from each of these sites have a characteristic morphology and rate.

Ectopic beats can occur in isolation or in series, when they are referred to as *couplets, triplets* or *salvos* (if four or more). Alternatively, they may occur every second or third beat, when they are known as *bigeminy* or *trigeminy*.

In terms of aetiology, ectopic rhythms occur either due to increased excitability or 'automaticity' of a group of cardiac cells, or as an escape rhythm in response to a slow intrinsic heart rate.

Ectopic beats are usually a benign phenomenon. They are found almost universally in the general population, and are well tolerated. Rarely, they cause significant symptoms and/ or represent serious underlying pathology, but in the vast majority of cases reassurance is all that is required.

6.1 Atrial ectopic beats (Figure 6.1)

Key features

- Normal sinus beats are interspersed with PQRS ① complexes occurring earlier than expected
- The P wave is often small, and the PR interval short ② The following normal sinus beat occurs later than expected ③
- The morphology of the QRS complex is the same as in sinus rhythm.

Pathophysiology

P waves are generated from a focus in the atrium other than the SA node. Because of this, the morphology of the P waves is different. If atrial premature beats all arise from one focus, all the ectopic P waves will look alike. If there are several foci throughout the atrial myocardium, each P wave will look different, and the PR interval will be of different lengths. This is known as *wandering atrial pacemaker*.

Clinical relevance

Atrial ectopic beats are usually a normal finding. Other causes are SA node disease, structural atrial disease, ischaemic heart disease, increased parasympathetic activity, electrolyte disturbance and drugs.

Management

Most individuals are asymptomatic and require no further investigation or treatment. Care should be taken not to confuse this condition with atrial fibrillation, as the two are managed quite differently.

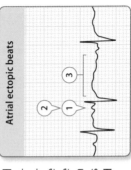

Atrial ectopic beats

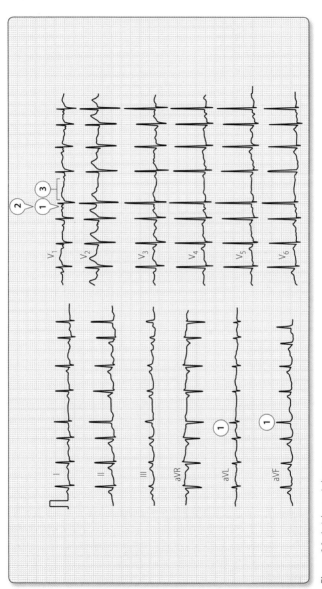

Figure 6.1 Atrial ectopic beats.

6.2 Ventricular ectopic beats (Figure 6.2)

Key features

- Normal sinus beats (N) are interspersed with broad QRS complexes occurring earlier than expected ①
- Each extra, or 'ectopic', beat is followed by a full compensatory pause ②
- Ectopic QRS complexes appear different from the sinus beat QRS complexes – they are broader and have a different axis
- If all ectopic beats look alike they are known as *unifocal*, if are do not all look alike they are known as *multifocal*

Pathophysiology

A number of mechanisms can cause ventricular ectopic beats. Usually a ventricular myocyte depolarises spontaneously. In other cases electrolyte disturbance or drug toxicity can trigger ectopics. Ventricular scarring from previous myocardial infarction is a third possible cause.

Clinical relevance

Ventricular ectopic beats are found in normal individuals and are usually asymptomatic. Some experience palpitations, rarely ventricular ectopics can be due to underlying heart disease.

Management

Excluding and treating any underlying heart disease is the priority. In highly symptomatic patients anti-arrhythmic drugs or catheter ablation can be used to suppress ectopics.

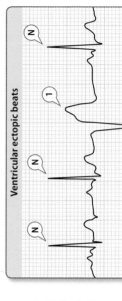

Ventricular ectopic beats

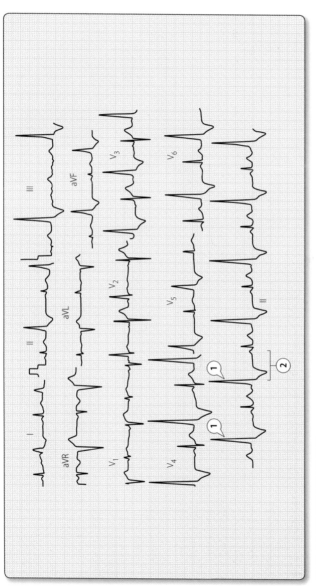

Figure 6.2 Ventricular ectopic beats.

6.3 Junctional ectopic beats (Figure 6.3)

Key features

- Normal sinus beats are interspersed with QRS complexes occurring earlier than expected ①
- The premature QRS complexes have the same morphology as in sinus rhythm, but are not preceded by a P wave ②
- There may be a P wave immediately after the QRS complex or buried in the QRS complex itself ③
- The following normal sinus beat occurs later than expected

Pathophysiology

Depolarisation starts from at or just below the AV node. As this propagates from the node down the His–Purkinje system the QRS morphology is normal. At the same time, the impulse propagates up to the atrium, resulting in the atrial depolarisation (P wave) occurring simultaneously or just after the QRS. As a result, the P wave may be hidden in the QRS complex or immediately after it.

Clinical relevance

Usually benign, they can be triggered by increased sympathomimetic levels, including physiological stress due to illness or electrolyte disturbance. They can occur as an escape rhythm in the setting of sinus pause or sinus bradycardia (see sinus pause, Section 4.2).

Management

Most individuals are asymptomatic, and junctional ectopic beats are a benign or normal finding. Associated bradycardia or sinus pause should be investigated and treated.

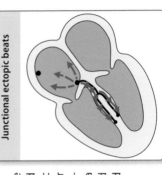

Junctional ectopic beats

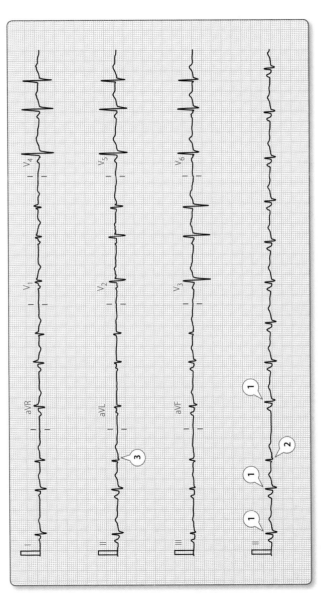

Figure 6.3 Junctional ectopic beats.

Atrial arrhythmias

Abnormal heart rhythms arising from the atria occur by a variety of mechanisms, including ectopy (see Chapter 6) and re-entry (see Chapter 8). However, the most common atrial arrhythmia is atrial fibrillation (AF), the aetiology of which is poorly understood, but probably includes elements of both re-entry and enhanced automaticity.

As with most arrhythmias, the main determinant of symptoms and signs is overall ventricular rate. The choice of treatment, and the urgency with which it must be delivered is therefore largely guided by the patient's clinical status.

In certain atrial arrhythmias, however, there is an increased risk of stroke, which must be taken into account in determining the best management plan for the patients.

Automatic-focus and scar re-entry atrial tachycardia

7.1   Atrial tachycardia (Figure 7.1)

Key features

- Regular P waves with a constant rate > 100 beats/min ①
- P wave has unusual morphology ②
- P wave may be conducted in a 1:1 or 2:1 ratio

Pathophysiology

The atrium depolarises in a regular manner, but the depolarisation arises from a site other than the sinus node (**SN**), which is suppressed. This can be due to one of two mechanisms. There may be an automatic focus (**A**) in the atrium that spontaneously depolarises in the same way as for atrial ectopic beats, but at a more rapid rate. In re-entry forms, scarring allows depolarisation to re-enter the atrial network (**B**). Both pathologies lead to higher atrial and overall heart rates.

Clinical relevance

Atrial tachycardia is often symptomatic due to the rapid rate, but is not life threatening. It may occur in the setting of a normal heart if it is automatic in origin. Scar-related re-entrant AT can be a sign of underlying hypertension, ischaemia, cardiomyopathy or post-procedural scarring.

Management

An acute episode may be terminated by drugs or DC cardioversion. Drugs or radiofrequency ablation may prevent recurrences.

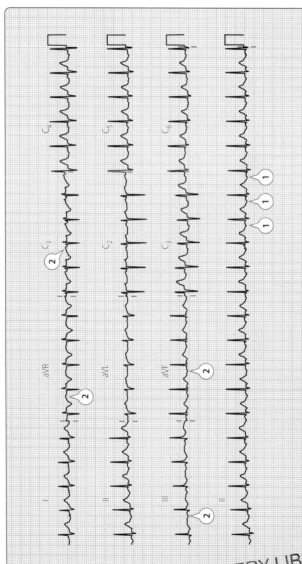

Figure 7.1 Atrial tachycardia.

7.2 Multifocal atrial tachycardia (Figure 7.2)

Key features

- Ventricular rate > 90–100 beats/min ①
- A P wave precedes every QRS complex ②
- Three or more types of P wave are seen, with different morphology, axis and PR interval
- QRS complexes may occur irregularly, but are morphologically identical to sinus rhythm

Pathophysiology

When the atria are damaged or distended, the foci of atrial myocytes can spontaneously depolarise at rates higher than that of the sinus node. Under sympathetic stimulation this rate of depolarisation increases, and a tachycardia ensues, with impulses from the various foci being transmitted through to the ventricles.

Clinical relevance

Patients may experience palpitations, breathlessness or chest tightness, or may be asymptomatic. If the tachycardia is not detected and continues for a long time, the heart muscle may weaken (tachycardia-mediated cardiomyopathy). Care should be taken not to confuse this condition with AF, where no discernible P waves are seen, or atrial flutter, where there is continuous uniform atrial activity.

Management

Drug therapy (e.g. beta blockers or verapamil) can be used to suppress atrial ectopy and control the ventricular rate. If this fails to control the ventricular rate the atrioventricular (AV) node can be ablated and a pacemaker implanted.

Clinical insight

If the ventricular rate is less than 100 beats/min the rhythm is called 'wandering atrial pacemaker' – the pacemaker site shifts between the SA node, the atria, and/or the AV node

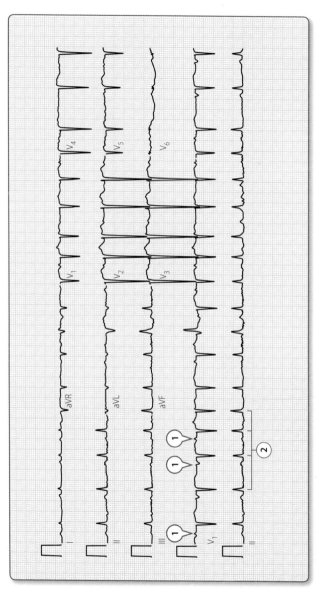

Figure 7.2 Multifocal atrial tachycardia.

7.3   Atrial flutter (Figure 7.3)

Key features

- 'Saw-tooth' appearance of baseline ①
- Ventricular rate can be fast, normal or slow, and may be regular or irregular ②

Pathophysiology

In atrial flutter there is a large or 'macro' re-entrant circuit in one of the atria. In *typical* atrial flutter, as shown here, the circuit is around the right atrium from top to bottom, at a rate of 300 beats/min, or one large square. Because the majority of electrical activity is travelling towards and away from the inferior leads, this is where the flutter waves are seen best. Like in AF, the AV node does not keep up with the fast atrial rate, often transmitting every other, or every third, atrial signal (2:1 and 3:1, respectively).

Clinical relevance

Like AF, people with atrial flutter may be symptomatic or asymptomatic, and the heart rate may be fast, slow or normal. There is an increased risk of stroke as compared with the normal population.

Management

The management of atrial flutter is similar to that of AF with stroke prevention, and measures to control the ventricular rate and/or maintain sinus rhythm.

DC cardioversion is an alternative to drugs for restoring sinus rhythm during an episode. Radiofrequency ablation of atrial flutter is often highly effective in preventing recurrence.

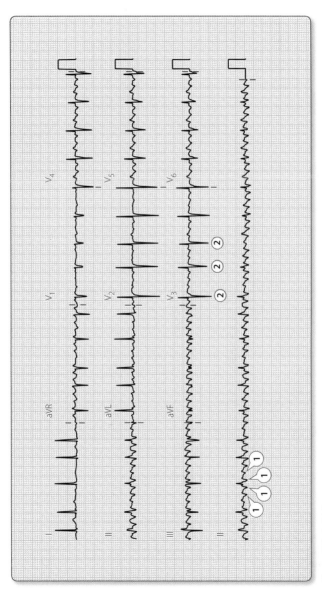

Figure 7.3 Atrial flutter

7.4 Atrial fibrillation (Figure 7.4)

Key features

- Irregularly irregular QRS complexes ①
- Chaotic baseline – no clear P waves ②
- QRS complex looks normal, or the same as when the patient is in sinus rhythm

Pathophysiology

Scar or distension of the atria predisposes to disordered atrial activity. This leads to very fast, irregular atrial contraction known as 'fibrillation'. The AV node regulates transmission of these signals to the ventricles resulting in slower, but still irregular ventricular contraction.

Clinical relevance

Atrial contraction, which is compromised in AF, contributes around 20% of ventricular filling, the rest being passive. Most patients are therefore asymptomatic, provided the rate is well controlled. Some may feel tired, breathless or unwell. The loss of regular, smooth blood flow through the left atrium can predispose to clot formation. This, in turn, increases the risk of stroke.

Management

During an acute episode, sinus rhythm can be restored either by drugs, or by DC cardioversion. In the longer term ventricular rate, or less commonly rhythm, can be controlled by drugs. If this fails electrical interventions may be considered. Atrial fibrillation is associated with an increased risk of stroke, and most patients should therefore be treated with anticoagulants.

Clinical insight

- If you are not sure whether the QRS complexes are irregular or not, get a piece of paper and mark where the R waves fall. Move the piece of paper along the baseline to see if any pattern can be found. If not, this is very likely to be AF.
- Early in AF the baseline can be very chaotic and you may think P waves are visible. If you are not sure, compare different 'P waves'. If they truly are P waves they should all look alike, and the PR interval should be regular. Later on, the baseline becomes less obviously chaotic, and can even look flat.

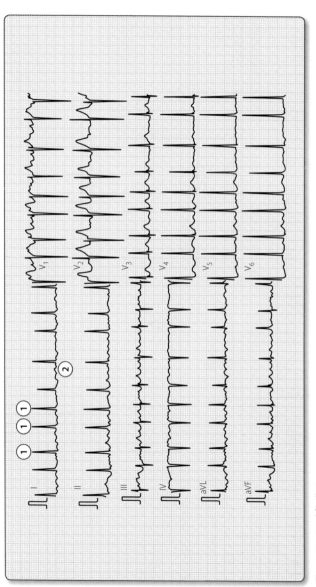

Figure 7.4 Atrial fibrillation.

7.5   Atrial fibrillation with left bundle branch block (Figure 7.5)

Key features

- Irregularly irregular broad complex tachycardia ①
- No discernible P waves/fibrillatory waves ②
- The morphology of the QRS complex is a typical bundle branch block pattern

Pathophysiology

AF and bundle branch block may coexist, giving the appearance of broad complex tachycardia. The QRS complexes are irregularly irregular, as would be expected in AF.

Clinical relevance

The main diagnostic dilemma with this rhythm is distinguishing it from ventricular tachycardia. The diagnosis is made on the basis of the irregular nature and the typical bundle branch block QRS pattern.

Management

The management is as for the underlying rhythm of AF. The patient should be assessed for risk of stroke and given anticoagulation medication as necessary. Drug therapy or ablation may be needed either to control the ventricular response rate or to restore and maintain sinus rhythm.

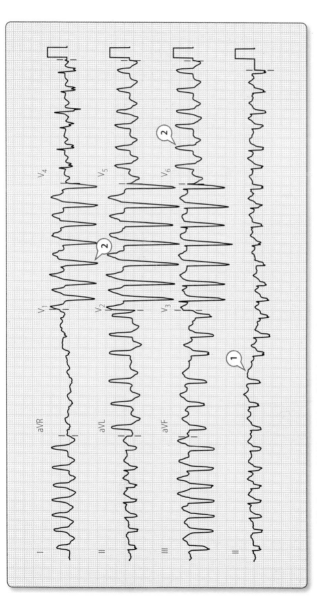

Figure 7.5 Atrial fibrillation with left bundle branch block.

chapter 8

Narrow-complex tachyarrhythmias (supraventricular tachycardias)

The narrow-complex tachyarrhythmias described here, commonly referred to as the supraventricular tachycardias (SVTs), are all due to the presence of an abnormal conducting pathway in the heart. Under certain circumstances, electrical signals are able to travel down the normal conducting pathway, and then go back up an abnormal pathway, or vice versa, and then continue around this loop. This phenomenon is known as *re-entry*.

Like other tachyarrhythmias, the patient's response depends largely on the heart rate and the duration of the arrhythmia. Fortunately, in the majority of cases the arrhythmia is readily terminated with drugs, and in the long term may be amenable to radiofrequency ablation, during which the abnormal pathway is identified and destroyed.

8.1   Atrioventricular nodal re-entrant tachycardia (Figure 8.1)

Key features

- QRS rate >100 beats/min
- QRS axis and morphology are similar to when in sinus rhythm - complexes are narrow unless there is coexisting bundle branch block
- No clear P waves
- R'/notching of QRS complex in V_1 ①

Pathophysiology

Two AV nodal pathways are present, and the re-entrant circuit utilises the fast and slow pathways of the AV node itself.

During tachycardia there is near simultaneous activation of the atria and ventricles during tachycardia. This results in there being no clear P waves, as they are buried within the QRS complex. Often there may be an R'/notching of the QRS complex in V_1 due to the concealed P wave.

Clinical relevance

AV nodal re-entrant tachycardia is the commonest type of SVT. It is not associated with structural heart disease. It results in palpitations, breathlessness and, potentially, syncope.

Management

A bolus of IV adenosine will terminate the tachycardia by temporarily blocking the AV node. Alternative drugs include beta blockers or calcium channel blockers. Radiofrequency ablation can offer a long term cure.

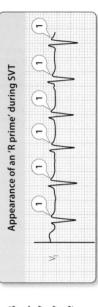

Appearance of an 'R prime' during SVT

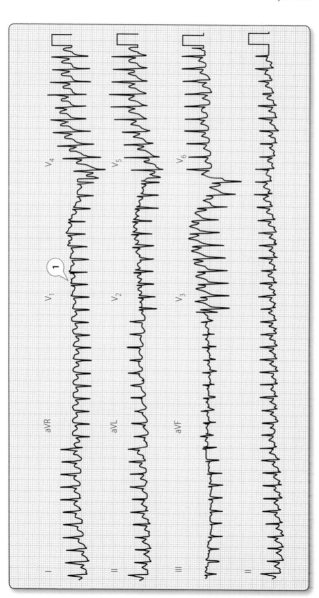

Figure 8.1 Atrioventricular nodal re-entrant tachycardia.

8.2 Atrioventricular reciprocating tachycardia (Figure 8.2)

Key features

- QRS rate >100 beats/min
- QRS axis and morphology are usually the same as when in sinus rhythm ①
- A retrograde P wave is usually seen shortly after the QRS complex ②
- QRS alternans may be present ③

Pathophysiology

In atrioventricular reciprocating tachycardia (AVRT) an extra or 'accessory' pathway joins the atria and ventricles. This allows 're-entry' of the depolarisation wave from the ventricles to the atria (causing the retrograde P wave seen on the ECG), and the circuit begins again.

Clinical relevance

AVRT is the second most common form of SVT and is usually not associated with structural heart disease. It may exist as Wolff–Parkinson–White syndrome (i.e. with pre-excitation) or it may be "concealed".

Management

As with AVNRT, adenosine (or another anti-arrhythmic) and radiofrequency ablation are the main treatment options.

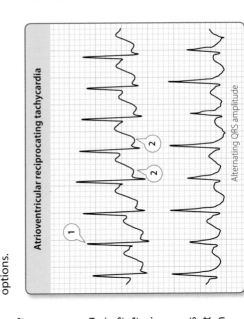

Atrioventricular reciprocating tachycardia

Alternating QRS amplitude

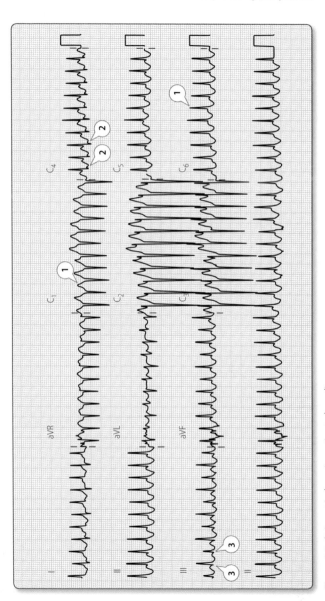

Figure 8.2 Atrioventricular reciprocating tachycardia.

8.3 Wolff–Parkinson–White syndrome: right-sided pathway (Figure 8.3)

Key features

- Short PR interval (< 120 ms) ①
- Delta wave, slurred onset of QRS complex ②
- Broad QRS complex ③
- Negative delta wave in V_1 and leftward axis locates pathway as right lateral (right free wall) ④

Pathophysiology

In WPW syndrome there is an accessory pathway connecting the atrium to the ventricle. This accessory pathway allows early depolarisation of part of the ventricle just before normal depolarisation via the His-Purkinje system giving the appearance of the delta wave and short PR interval. The location and shape of the delta wave allows cardiologists to predict the location of the accessory pathway.

Clinical relevance

The presence of the accessory pathway makes re-entry possible, putting the patient at risk of AVRT- type supraventricular tachycardia (see 8.2). More seriously, if AF occurs this can be conducted rapidly via the accessory pathway to the ventricles putting the patient at risk of VF.

Management

In symptomatic or high-risk patients radiofrequency ablation is the treatment of choice.

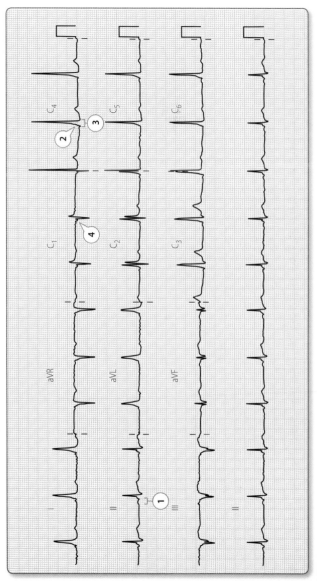

Figure 8.3 Wolff–Parkinson–White syndrome: right-sided pathway.

8.4   Wolff–Parkinson–White syndrome: left lateral pathway (Figure 8.4)

Key features

- Short PR interval <120 ms ①
- Delta wave, slurred onset of QRS complex ②
- Broad QRS complex ③
- Positive delta wave in V_1 and a negative delta wave in I/aVL locates the pathway to the lateral or 'free wall' of the left ventricle ④

Pathophysiology

There is an accessory pathway connecting the atria and ventricles, in this case at the lateral or 'free' wall of the left ventricle. The early activation of the ventricle via the accessory pathway is known as 'pre-excitation' and is seen on the ECG as a delta wave with a short PR interval.

Clinical relevance

The patient could be at risk of SVT (AVRT type, see Section 8.2). This may present as palpitations, breathlessness or lightheadedness. Syncope is a worrying feature and should be investigated further.

Management

Patients with an accessory pathway (as in WPW) may undergo an electrophysiological study in order to determine how fast the pathway can conduct electrical signals from the atria to the ventricles. In high-risk or symptomatic individuals, radiofrequency ablation is the treatment of choice.

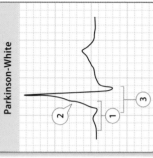

ECG features of Wolff-Parkinson-White

Broad complex tachyarrhythmias

Broad QRS complexes occur for one of two reasons: either the rhythm arises in the ventricle, as in ventricular tachycardia (VT), or the rhythm arises in the atria and is aberrantly transmitted to the ventricles, for example due to bundle branch block or via an accessory pathway (SVT with aberrancy).

Ventricular arrhythmias are most commonly a manifestation of ischaemic heart disease and may be fatal. Ventricular fibrillation, for example, is incompatible with life, and requires immediate defibrillation. The degree to which other forms of VT are tolerated depends largely on the heart rate and left ventricular function. These also frequently require cardioversion or defibrillation.

Aberrantly conducted supraventricular arrhythmias are generally less likely to cause haemodynamic compromise than ventricular arrhythmias and are managed according to the underlying supraventricular rhythm.

Determining the difference between ventricular arrhythmias and aberrantly conducted supraventricular arrhythmias can be difficult, even for the expert. In the acute situation, however, the principles of management are the same, including assessing the patient's haemodynamic status and, if compromised, delivering rapid cardioversion. In more stable patients a trial of anti-arrhythmic drugs and/or treatment of the underlying condition may be attempted in the first instance.

9.1 Monomorphic ventricular tachycardia (Figure 9.1)

Key features

- QRS complex rate is >100 beats/min
- QRS complex is broad > 120 ms ①
- Onset of the R wave is slurred ②
- Signs of atrioventricular (AV) dissociation ③
- QRS complex morphology is constant

Pathophysiology

Scarred ventricle tissue acts as a site for re-entry. This continuous, short circuit of activation (**A**) propagates out from the scar across the remaining ventricle tissue (**B**). As the depolarisation does not spread via the usual His–Purkinje pathway, it is slow and results in a slurred onset broad QRS complex. The depolarisation propagates away from the scar, and has a bizarre morphology and axis.

Clinical relevance

VT is usually a sign of scarring processes affecting the ventricle. The most common causes are ischaemic heart disease, cardiomyopathy and surgery. VT is a potentially life-threatening arrhythmia and can rapidly result in cardiac arrest.

Management

Standard adult life support algorithms should be followed in the acute setting, including DC cardioversion. Many patients will require an implantable defibrillator in the long term. Underlying disease processes must be addressed (e.g. revascularisation for ischaemic heart disease).

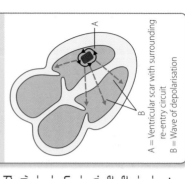

Ventricular scar as a focus for VT

A = Ventricular scar with surrounding re-entry circuit
B = Wave of depolarisation

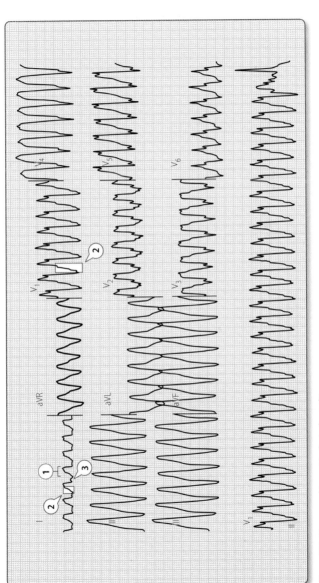

Figure 9.1 Monomorphic ventricular tachycardia.

9.2 Polymorphic ventricular tachycardia (Figure 9.2)

Key features

- QRS complexes are broad and morphologically different to those in sinus rhythm
- QRS complex rate is >100 beats/min
- QRS complex morphology varies ①
- RR interval varies ②
- Dissociated P waves may be present ③
- Capture or fusion beats may be seen (as in monomorphic VT)
- QRS complex morphology changes from beat to beat

Pathophysiology

Polymorphic ventricular tachycardia (PMVT) occurs when there is an abnormal focus of electrical activity in the ventricular myocardium. The pattern of depolarisation often varies randomly and results in varying QRS morphology and RR interval. Unlike the torsade de pointes form of VT there is no predictable or recognisable pattern to the changing QRS morphology. The most common reasons for the occurrence of PMVT are acute ischaemia, electrolyte disturbance or hereditary conditions (see long QT and Brugada syndromes, Sections 11.3 and 11.4).

Clinical relevance

VT is a life-threatening arrhythmia. It is usually poorly tolerated by the patient and rapidly degenerates into ventricular fibrillation with associated cardiac arrest.

Management

Urgent cardioversion or defibrillation is required to restore sinus rhythm. Advanced life-support protocols should be followed for other acute supportive measures. The underlying cause (ischaemia or electrolyte imbalance) should be corrected. Many patients will ultimately need implantation of a cardiac defibrillator.

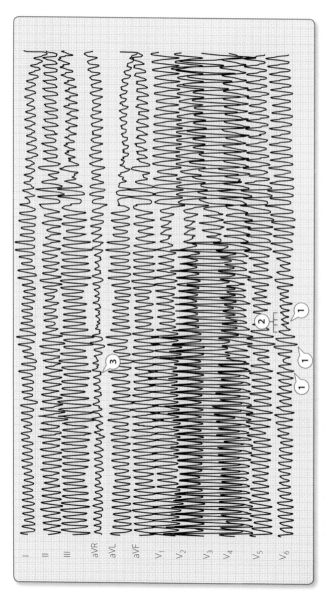

Figure 9.2 Polymorphic ventricular tachycardia.

9.3 Torsade de pointes (Figure 9.3)

Key features

- Regular, broad QRS complexes ①
- Rapidly changing axis and QRS morphology ②
- 'R on T' phenomenon at the onset of tachycardia ③

Pathophysiology

Torsade de pointes (or 'twisting of the points') is a form of VT associated with congenital or acquired long QT segment syndromes. The long QT segment reflects a long refractory and repolarisation time. If a ventricular premature beat falls within this refractory period, it can be superimposed on the T wave of the preceding normal sinus beat. This is known as the 'R on T' phenomenon, and can precipitate ventricular arrhythmias (in this case torsade de pointes).

Clinical relevance

Patients may present with palpitations, dizziness, breathlessness, chest pain or syncope. The degree to which the arrhythmia is tolerated depends largely on the underlying ventricular function.

Management

Torsade de pointes is generally a rapid and haemodynamically unstable rhythm, and requires cardioversion. If the condition is well tolerated, correction of reversible causes (e.g. electrolyte disturbance) may terminate the arrhythmia. In all cases, an underlying cause should be sought and corrected.

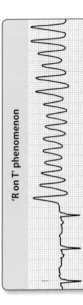

'R on T' phenomenon

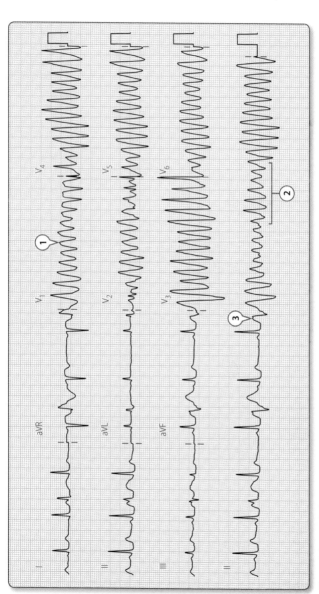

Figure 9.3 Torsade de pointes.

9.4 Ventricular fibrillation (Figure 9.4)

Key features

- Completely chaotic recording in all 12 ECG leads
- As ventricular fibrillation continues the QRS complexes get smaller, until eventually the ECG recording has the appearance of asystole

Pathophysiology

Completely disordered electrical activity in the ventricles causes them to 'fibrillate'. The fibrillating ventricle is said to look like a 'bag of worms'. Neither ventricular filling nor ventricular systole can occur, and cardiac arrest ensues.

Clinical relevance

VF is not compatible with a cardiac output and is a cause of cardiac arrest. Cardiac ischaemia is the most common cause, with electrolyte imbalance, drugs, pulmonary embolus and chest trauma being among many other causes.

Care should be taken not to mistake electrical interference for VF. A VF patient will likely lose consciousness in the time it takes to check the electrical connections.

Management

In the context of a witnessed cardiac arrest a precordial thump may be attempted. DC cardioversion is the most effective treatment for restoring sinus rhythm, and may be used in conjunction with antiarrhythmic drugs (e.g. amiodarone). Unfortunately, many people will not survive a VF cardiac arrest.

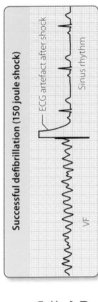

Successful defibrillation (150 joule shock)

ECG artefact after shock

Sinus rhythm

VF

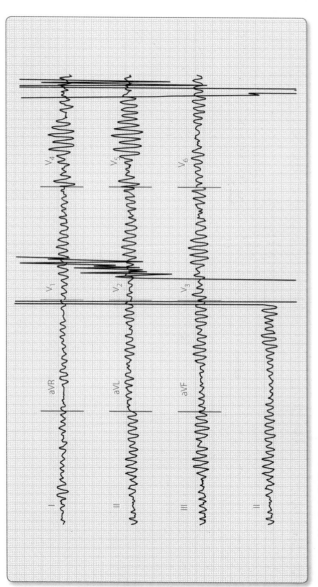

Figure 9.4 Ventricular fibrillation.

9.5   Supraventricular tachycardia with bundle branch block (Figure 9.5)

Key features

- Regular, broad QRS complex
- Precordial leads are *not* concordant, i.e. there is progression of the R wave from V_1 through to V_6 (positive to negative in right bundle branch block (BBB), and negative to positive in left BBB), resembling a typical BBB pattern
- Axis is usually normal ①
- P waves usually seen (no AV dissociation, e.g. capture and fusion beats) ②

Pathophysiology

Supraventricular tachycardia (SVT) and bundle branch block may coexist, giving the appearance of broad QRS complex tachycardia. The BBB may be present in sinus rhythm, or it may be rate-dependent, occurring only during the tachycardia.

Clinical relevance

The main diagnostic dilemma with this rhythm is distinguishing it from VT. While careful analysis of the ECG will often yield the answer, in an unstable patient or when the diagnosis is uncertain, the patient can be managed safely, irrespective of the electrical diagnosis.

Management

In the unstable patient, prompt cardioversion is the correct treatment for any tachyarrhythmia, irrespective of the underlying diagnosis. Older age, cardiac risk factors and the presence of known ischemic heart disease make VT more likely, and the patient should be treated as such. In the absence of these factors, and in patients with a known diagnosis of SVT with BBB, adenosine can be used either to terminate the tachyarrhythmia (if the SVT is AV re-entrant tachycardia or AV nodal re-entrant tachycardia), or to unmask the underlying atrial rhythm (as in atrial flutter or atrial tachycardia).

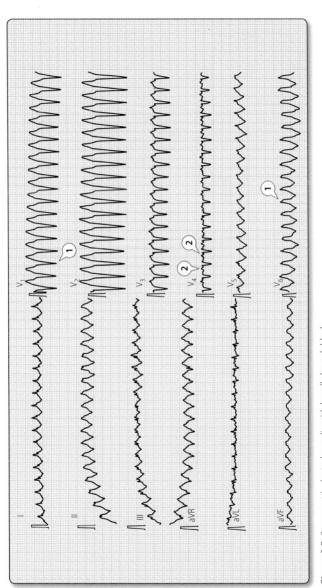

Figure 9.5 Supraventricular tachycardia with bundle branch block.

Ischaemia and infarction

It is important to be able to recognise the ECG manifestations of cardiac ischaemia and myocardial infarction (MI) as they represent important pathology that often needs urgent treatment. Coronary artery disease underlies a range of clinical conditions, from stable angina through unstable angina and non-ST segment elevation MI (NSTEMI), to acute ST segment elevation MI (STEMI). Ischaemic heart disease may also manifest as cardiac arrhythmias.

Stable angina occurs when coronary atheroma restricts the flow of blood down the coronary arteries. During exercise or stress, when myocardial oxygen demand is higher, this restricted blood supply may be temporarily insufficient, leading to ischaemia of the subendocardial myocardium (the part of heart muscle furthest away from the coronary artery). If an ECG is recorded during one of these episodes it will often show transient changes, including ST segment depression or T wave inversion, or it may be normal.

Similar ECG changes may be seen during unstable angina or a NSTEMI but, unlike stable angina, the symptoms and ECG abnormalities do not predictably occur on exertion, with associated relief at rest. Unstable angina and NSTEMI are distinguished by a rise in cardiac enzymes. However, this rise might not be detectable for up to 12 hours after the onset of symptoms, and thus the initial evaluation and treatment are essentially identical.

STEMI occurs when one or more coronary arteries becomes acutely critically narrowed or occluded. Myocytes through the full thickness of the ventricular wall are damaged by ischaemia. This is a medical emergency and requires urgent treatment to restore blood supply to the affected myocardium in order to minimise the risk of heart failure or death. While ST elevation is recognised as the hallmark of STEMI, the ECG changes vary, and evolve over time:

- Very early in the process the ST segment may be only minimally elevated, but T waves are tall and/or pointed (so-called 'hyperacute' T waves).
- In minutes to hours the ST segment becomes elevated. It is classically convex, or planar, but any elevated ST segment should be regarded with suspicion.
- In hours to days the ST segment settles, and T waves become inverted (or they may be biphasic or flattened).
- In the long term, the presence of Q waves and T wave inversion will often persist.

It should be noted that, while the changes seen in STEMI are specific to a territory of cardiac muscle, corresponding to the coronary artery supplying that territory, the same is usually not true for cardiac ischaemia.

Time dependent ECG changes due to acute myocardial infarction

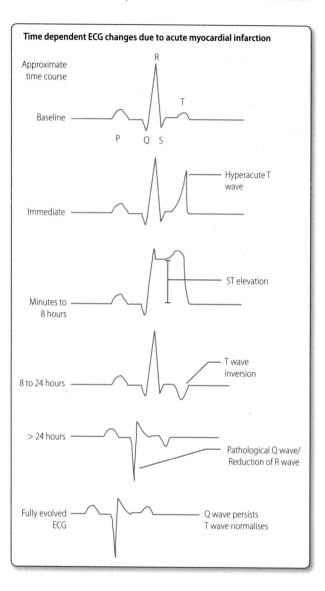

10.1 ST segment depression (cardiac ischaemia) (Figure 10.1)

Key features

- ST segment depression in lateral leads ①
- ST segment may be downsloping or planar ②
- Upsloping ST segment depression is less suggestive of ischaemia

Pathophysiology

Ischaemia alters the transmembrane potential of cardiac myocytes, and affects the shape and duration of the action potential. The difference in electrical properties between ischaemic and normal zones of the myocardium creates a voltage gradient between them, a so-called *injury current*. This is seen as ST segment deviations: transmural ischaemia causes ST elevation, whereas ischaemia confined to the subendocardium shows as ST depression.

Clinical relevance

Patients with cardiac ischaemia will usually experience chest pain and/or breathlessness. When these symptoms occur on exertion and are relieved by rest they represent stable angina. If symptoms are severe, becoming more frequent or occurring at rest an acute coronary syndrome or MI may occur, and is a medical emergency.

Management

Stable angina can be treated with anti-anginal medication (e.g. nitrates or calcium channel blockers). Patients should be assessed for risk of future MI and started on preventive medication. Those with acute ischaemia should be managed on a coronary care unit with antiplatelet agents, anti-anginals and opiates as needed. High-risk patients should be considered for coronary angiography with a view to revascularisation.

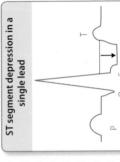

ST segment depression in a single lead

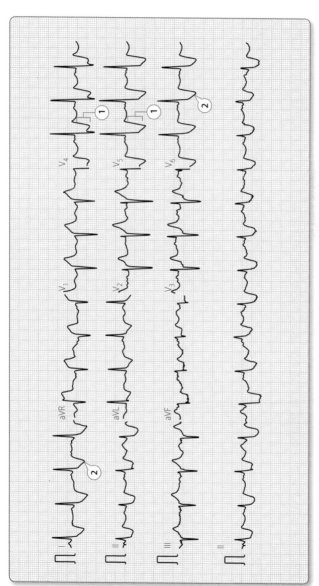

Figure 10.1 ST segment depression (cardiac ischaemia).

10.2 Acute myocardial ischaemia: T wave inversion and the LAD syndrome (Figure 10.2)

Key features

- Deep, symmetrical 'arrowhead' T wave inversion in the anterior or anterolateral leads ①
- ST segment depression may also be present ②

Pathophysiology

Acute ischaemia in the territory of the lateral anterior descending (LAD) artery is seen as T wave inversion in the affected leads. This represents abnormal repolarisation of the myocardium.

Clinical relevance

There are many causes of T wave inversion, and it is normal in some leads on the ECG. It is relatively non-specific for ischaemia unless it is deep and symmetrical. T wave inversion is considered abnormal in leads V_3–V_6, II and aVF. Causes of deep, symmetrical T wave inversion include myocardial ischaemia, MI, hypertro-

phic cardiomyopathy, juvenile pattern or intracranial haemorrhage.

Management

The ECG must be interpreted in the clinical context. In the presence of acute cardiac ischaemia or infarction, measures should be taken to relieve pain and improve coronary blood flow (i.e. opiate analgesia and nitrates), antiplatelet therapy should be given, and consideration should be given to early coronary angiography with a view to percutaneous coronary intervention.

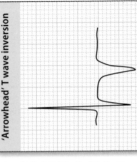

'Arrowhead' T wave inversion

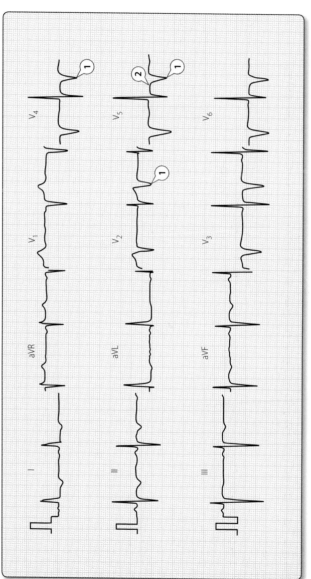

Figure 10.2 Acute myocardial ischaemia: T wave inversion and the LAD syndrome.

10.3 ST segment elevation myocardial infarction: anterior (Figure 10.3)

Key features

- Widespread ST elevation in the anterolateral leads (some or all of V_1–V_6, I, II, and aVL) [1]
- 'Reciprocal' ST depression may be seen in other leads [2]
- ST elevation in aVR may suggest left main stem involvement

Pathophysiology

The anterolateral wall of the heart is supplied by the LAD artery. When blood flow down this artery is severely compromised, ST segment elevation MI occurs.

Clinical relevance

While all ST segment elevation MIs are serious cardiological emergencies, widespread infarctions affecting the anterolateral wall can be particularly dangerous, as the left ventricle loses its blood supply and pumps more weakly, leading to pulmonary oedema, low blood pressure and cardiogenic shock. Ventricular arrhythmias can occur and may cause cardiac arrest.

Management

Urgent reperfusion therapy, with percutaneous conary intervention or thrombolysis should be undertaken as early as possible. In the early stages, antiarrhythmic therapy or measures to support the left ventricle may be needed. In the longer term, the left ventricle should be studied echocardiographically to assess the degree of damage, and the need for any further treatments.

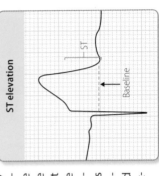

ST elevation

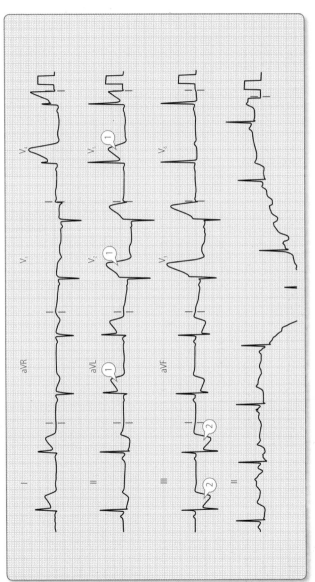

Figure 10.3 ST segment elevation myocardial infarction: anterior.

10.4 ST segment elevation myocardial infarction: acute inferior (Figure 10.4)

Key features

- ST segment elevation in the inferior leads (II, III, aVF) ①
- Reciprocal changes may be seen in other leads ②
- Hyperacute T waves may be present in the acute stage of infarction ③
- If the right coronary artery is large and dominant, infarction may extend into posterior (as in this example, ④) or lateral (leads AVL, V_5 and V_6) territories ⑤

Pathophysiology

The right coronary artery (RCA) (or rarely the circumflex artery) supplies the inferior myocardium. Disruption of supply can lead to infarction, showing as ST elevation in inferior leads. Depending on individual anatomy, ischaemia may extend to the lateral (leads II, V_5, V_6) or posterior wall (see section 10.5).

Clinical relevance

STEMI is a medical emergency and has a high mortality if untreated. The RCA also supplies the conducting system, therefore bradyarrhythmias are a frequent complication.

Management

Urgent reperfusion with thrombolytic agents or percutaneous intervention with balloons and stents is required. Bradyarrhythmias may indicate drugs (e.g. atropine) or temporary pacing.

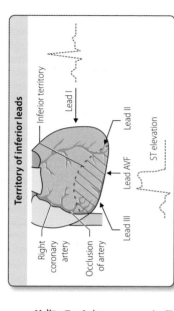

Territory of inferior leads

Inferior territory

Lead I

Lead II

Lead AVF

ST elevation

Lead III

Right coronary artery

Occlusion of artery

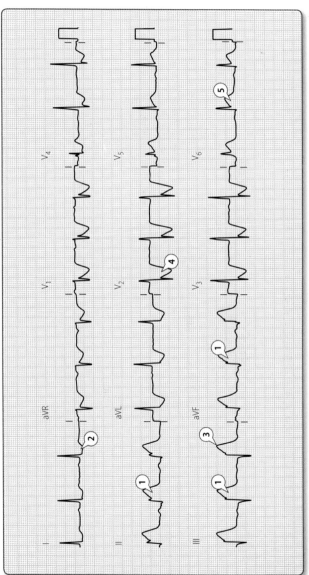

Figure 10.4 ST elevation inferior myocardial infarction (NB this patient also shows posterior extension of the infarction).

10.5 ST segment elevation myocardial infarction: posterior (Figure 10.5)

Key features

- ST segment depression in leads V_1, V_2 and V_3 ①
  If the ECG is inverted and looked at back to front, typical ST elevation can be seen in leads V_1, V_2 and V_3.
- Dominant R wave in leads V_1, V_2 and V_3 ②
- Possible inferior or lateral ST elevation depending on the individual's coronary anatomy ③
- Posterior leads V_7–V_9 will show ST elevation

Pathophysiology

Posterior MI is usually caused by a lesion in the circumflex artery supplying the back of the heart. Ordinarily there are no leads looking directly at the back of the heart, and thus a mirror image of a typical STEMI appearance is seen in the anterior leads – ST depression replaces ST elevation, and the dominant R wave replaces the Q wave.

Clinical relevance

Although more difficult to identify, posterior MI is as serious as anterior infarction.

Management

Urgent reperfusion therapy in the short term, and secondary prevention in the long term.

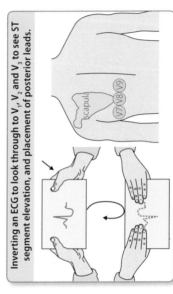

Inverting an ECG to look through to V_1, V_2 and V_3 to see ST segment elevation, and placement of posterior leads.

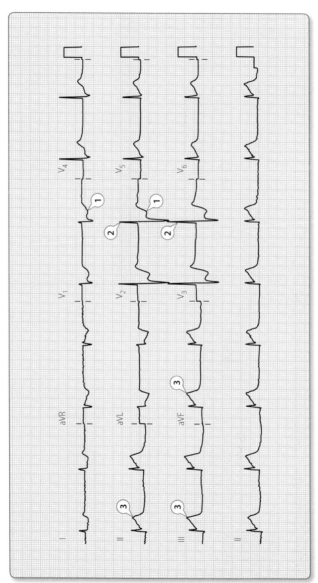

Figure 10.5 ST segment elevation myocardial Infarction: posterior.

10.6 Completed myocardial infarction (Figure 10.6)

Key features

- T wave inversion ①
- Resolution of previous ST segment elevation, with flattening or depression of the ST segment ②
- Fragmented appearance of the QRS complex ③
- Q waves present ④
- Small QRS complexes in chest leads with loss of normal R wave progression (normally negative in V_1 to positive in V_6) ⑤
- In a minority of cases the ECG may revert to normal

Pathophysiology

Post-MI ECG findings are variable, depending on the extent and territory of infarction, success or otherwise of reperfusion therapy, and the presence or absence of ventricular remodelling or conduction abnormalities.

Clinical relevance

No single ECG finding is specific for the previous MI, but ECG abnormalities relating to one specific area of myocardium must always raise that suspicion.

Management

Suspected undiagnosed previous MI should be further investigated in order to establish a diagnosis and institute appropriate secondary prevention. This includes medical therapy, lifestyle advice and an assessment of ventricular function.

Clinical insight

Definition of pathological Q waves:

- any Q wave in leads V_2 and V_3 > 20ms (half a small square)
- QS complex in leads V_2 and V_3 (complex with no R wave)
- any Q wave ≥ 30ms and ≥ 0.1 mV (1 small square) deep or a QS complex in leads I, II, AVL, AVF and V_4–V_6, present in two contiguous leads (two leads anatomically next to each other)
- the presence of a Q wave in V_1 or in lead III alone may be normal.

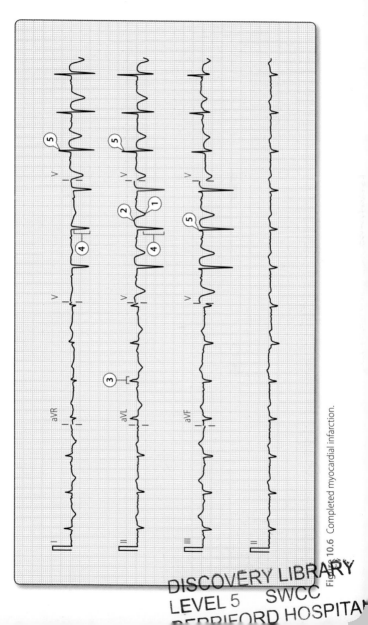

Figure 10.6 Completed myocardial infarction.

Inherited arrhythmia problems

chapter
11

The inherited cardiomyopathies are a group of diseases which can occur either spontaneously or by a variety of modes of inheritance. Genetic abnormalities can manifest in many ways, including abnormal gross anatomical development, disorders of myocyte organisation, abnormalities of the ion channels and predisposition to cardiac arrhythmias. There is often overlap between the above phenotypes, with certain genes being identified in the aetiology of a number of seemingly diverse conditions.

Inherited cardiomyopathies are manifest clinically as causes of right and/or left ventricular failure, or of cardiac arrhythmias, including sudden cardiac death. It is particularly important to identify the latter group of patients, as early detection can allow prophylactic measures to be taken and, if appropriate, allow family members to undergo screening.

A comprehensive review of all inherited cardiac disorders is beyond the scope of this text. The following examples serve merely to demonstrate some characteristic ECG patterns associated with important inherited cardiomyopathies, with a brief insight into the investigation and management of this diverse group of diseases.

11.1 Hypertrophic cardiomyopathy (Figure 11.1)

Key features

- Large-voltage QRS complexes and left axis deviation ①
- Associated ST segment and T wave changes ②
- Abnormal deep Q waves, especially in the inferior or septal leads ③
- Possible abnormal P waves

Pathophysiology

Increased ventricular mass is manifested by a large voltage QRS, and the ST–T wave abnormalities reflect subendocardial ischaemia. Q waves are caused by septal depolarisation of the hypertrophied myopathic muscle. Atrial enlargement is common and is manifested as abnormal P waves. Left axis deviation reflects the increased muscle mass of the left ventricle. In the apical variant of hypertrophic cardiomyopathy, deep T wave inversion may be seen in V_2–V_4.

Clinical relevance

Hypertrophic cardiomyopathy is a genetic condition with abnormal hypertrophy of the ventricular myocardium. Patients may present with chest pain, breathlessness or arrhythmia, or it may be an unexpected finding on the ECG or echocardiogram.

Management

Beta blockers or verapamil are often used to slow the heart rate, prolong diastole and improve ventricular filling. When hypertrophy of the septum impedes left ventricular outflow, surgical or percutaneous treatments can be used to reduce the ventricular mass. Patients at high risk of ventricular arrhythmias should be considered for an implantable cardiovertor defibrillator.

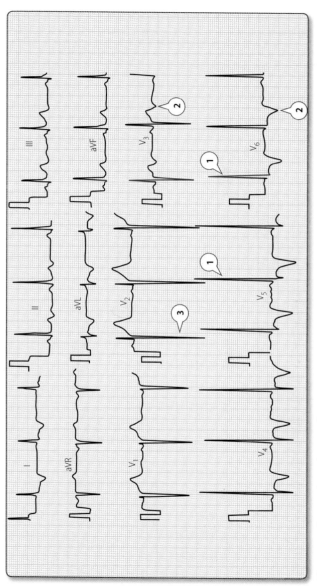

Figure 11.1 Hypertrophic cardiomyopathy.

11.2 Arrhythmogenic right ventricular dysplasia (Figure 11.2)

Key features

- Broad QRS, usually > 110 ms, with a second upward deflection in the right precordial leads (an *epsilon wave*), giving a right-bundle-branch-block-like appearance ①
- Possible associated T wave changes, usually in the right precordial leads ②

Pathophysiology

Arrhythmogenic right ventricular dysplasia (ARVD) is a cardiomyopathy that principally affects the right ventricle, and it is characterised by fibrofatty infiltration of the myocardium. ECG changes are therefore found principally in the right-sided leads (i.e. V₁, V₂, aVR). The epsilon wave reflects delayed activation of the right ventricular myocardium.

Clinical relevance

Fibrofatty infiltration of the myocardium leads to right ventricular thinning and dilatation. Despite this, clinical right ventricular failure is uncommon, and most patients present with symptomatic cardiac arrhythmias. These include frequent ventricular ectopic beats, and non-sustained or sustained ventricular tachycardia. It is an important cause of sudden cardiac death, especially in athletes.

Management

Because of the association between exercise and ventricular arrhythmia, patients with ARVD should not partake in competitive sports. Those at high risk of sudden death should receive an implantable cardiovertor defibrillator, with or without adjunctive drug therapy.

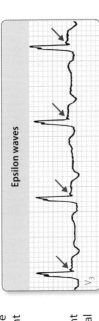

Epsilon waves

V₃

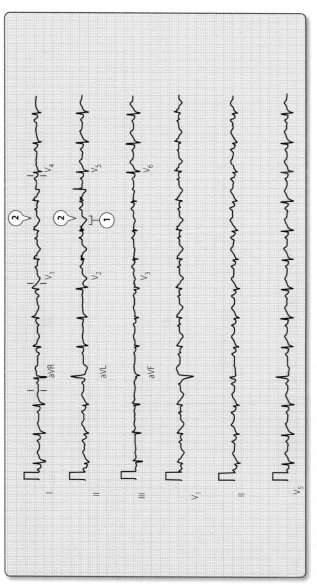

Figure 11.2 Arrhythmogenic right ventricular dysplasia.

11.3 Long QT syndrome (Figure 11.3)

Key features

- Corrected QT interval >440 ms ①
- Prominent U waves ②
- QT interval is best measured in leads V_2–V_3 and should be averaged over a number of beats ③

Pathophysiology

The QT interval is a measure of membrane repolarisation. The time required for repolarisation depends on the heart rate. At high heart rates the QT interval is longer, and this allows the heart muscle to repolarise fully before it is depolarised again. A normal corrected QT interval is <440 ms.

Clinical relevance

QT prolongation can be congenital or acquired. Acquired causes include drugs (particularly class 1A or 3 antiarrhythmic drugs, phenothiazines or tricyclic antidepressants), hypocalcaemia, hypothermia, cerebrovascular disease and cardiac ischaemia.

Congenital long QT syndromes are caused by genetic mutations of cardiac ion channels. Two main types are recognised clinically:

- Romano–Ward syndrome (autosomal-dominant inheritance and no deafness)
- Jervell–Lange–Nielsen syndrome (autosomal-recessive inheritance, associated with congenital deafness).

Long QT syndromes put patients at higher risk of torsade de pointes, a life-threatening arrhythmia.

Management

A reversible cause should be sought and treated. Care must always be taken when prescribing drugs for patients with long QT syndrome. In certain high-risk patients, implantable cardiovertor defibrillators can protect from sudden cardiac death.

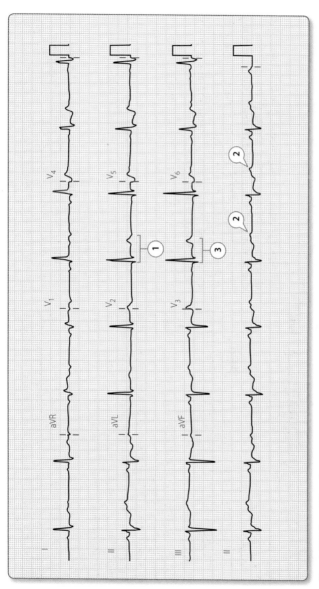

Figure 11.3 Long QT syndrome.

11.4 Brugada syndrome (Figure 11.4)

Key features

- Pseudo-right-bundle-branch-block appearance in V_1–V_3 ①
- ST elevation in leads V_1–V_3 ②
- ECG changes may be present all the time, may be transient, or may occur only when given provoking drugs.

The pattern of the ST elevation depends on the type of Brugada syndrome:

- Type 1: coved ST elevation > 2 mm, T wave inverted
- Type 2: saddle-shaped ST elevation > 2 mm, T wave positive or biphasic
- Type 3: saddle-shaped ST elevation < 2 mm, T wave positive

Pathophysiology

Brugada syndrome is an autosomal-dominant condition with variable expression. Various genes have been identified as possible causes, the best known of which is *SCN5A*, a gene that codes for cardiac sodium channels. The relationship between the ECG abnormalities and the genetic mutations is not fully understood, but it is thought to result from an abnormal action potential in certain myocytes.

Clinical relevance

There is an increased risk of ventricular and atrial arrhythmias. The diagnosis cannot be made on the ECG appearance alone, and

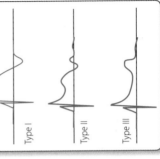

ST elevation pattern in V_1–V_3

Type I

Type II

Type III

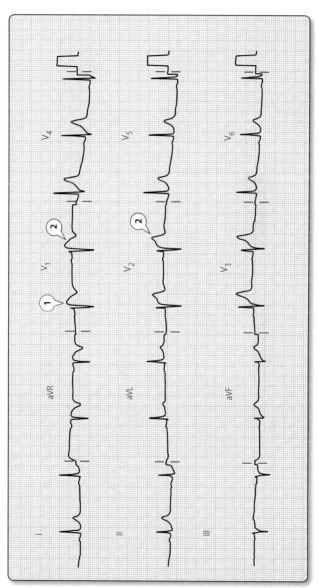

Figure 11.4 Brugada syndrome.

requires the presence of other features, such as documented ventricular arrhythmias, unexplained syncope or family history of sudden death.

Management

The mainstay of treatment is the prevention of sudden death from ventricular arrhythmias. There is no proven effective drug treatment, although quinidine and similar drugs may be useful. High-risk individuals, such as those with a prior history of cardiac arrest or unexplained syncope, should be considered for an implantable cardiovertor defibrillator.

Miscellaneous conditions

The range of cardiac and non-cardiac conditions that can be diagnosed by means of the ECG is vast, and cannot be covered in a single introductory text. Just as our knowledge of science and medicine is ever expanding, so too is our understanding of the ECG, with new original research still being published.

In the following chapter we consider a range of important conditions with characteristic ECG changes reflecting external physical or biochemical influences on the conducting system of the heart. By learning to recognise these patterns, valuable diagnostic information can be gleaned quickly and easily, at no risk to the patient.

12.1 Pericarditis (Figure 12.1)

Key features

- Concave 'saddle-shaped' ST segment elevation throughout the ECG ①
- T wave changes: T wave inversion, tall T waves (or they may be normal) ②
- PR segment depression ③

Pathophysiology

Pericarditis is inflammation of the pericardium. Potential causes include bacterial or viral infections, malignancy, collagen vascular disease, and post-operative or post-MI uraemia. When the adjacent epicardium is also affected, ECG changes are seen. The ST segment elevation reflects abnormal ventricular repolarisation. Abnormalities of the PR segment occur if the atria are affected. T wave changes are variable, again reflecting abnormalities of repolarisation, and may evolve acutely, similarly to myocardial infarction, or persist long term.

Clinical relevance

Acute pericarditis typically presents with chest pain, and may be mistaken for ST elevation MI. An associated pericardial effusion is often seen on echocardiogram.

Management

Idiopathic or viral pericarditis is usually self-limiting and can be treated with a course of non-steroidal anti-inflammatory drugs or aspirin, with or without colchicine. In cases where an alternative cause is found (e.g. uraemia), the cause should be addressed. Features suggesting a high risk of complications (e.g., high fever, presence of a large pericardial effusion, trauma, or elevated cardiac troponin), should prompt hospital admission.

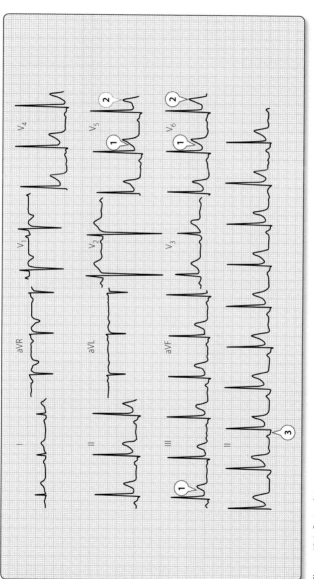

Figure 12.1 Pericarditis.

12.2 Left ventricular hypertrophy (Figure 12.2)

Key features

- Large-amplitude QRS complexes ①
- Slight widening of the QRS complex ②
- Delay in intrinsicoid deflection (the R wave peak time) – the upslope of the R wave is slightly slurred ③
- Possible associated left axis deviation
- Possible associated ST depression and/or T wave inversion (strain pattern) ④

Pathophysiology

Hypertrophy of the myocardium occurs either due to resistance to contraction, as in hypertension or aortic stenosis, or due to disease of the heart muscle itself, for example hypertrophic cardiomyopathy. The tall and wide QRS complex represents slower conduction through the large muscle mass, and the ST/T changes reflect subendocardial ischaemia.

Clinical relevance

LVH is associated with increased cardiovascular risk, including congestive cardiac failure, myocardial infarction, aortic root dilatation, stroke, ventricular arrhythmias and cardiac death. Correct identification and management can reduce these risks.

Management

Hypertension should be managed with lifestyle measures and, if necessary, medications. Other risk factors for cardiovascular disease should also be addressed.

Clinical insight

There are many different criteria for diagnosing LVH. The most commonly used are:

- S wave in V_1 + R wave in V_5 or V_6 $\geq$ 35 mm, and/or
- Large R wave in aVL >11 mm, or 18 mm if left axis deviation is present.

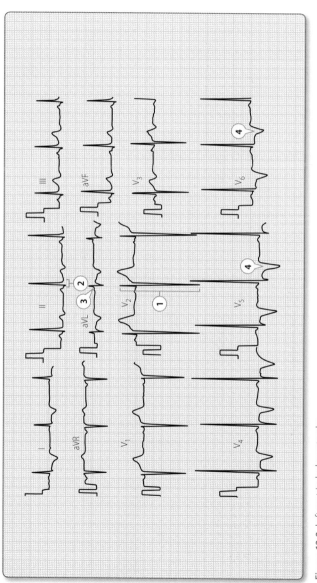

Figure 12.2 Left ventricular hypertrophy.

12.3 Right ventricular hypertrophy (Figure 12.3)

Key features

- Tall R wave in the right precordial leads (V_1 and V_2) ①
- Deep S wave in left precordial leads (V_5 and V_6) ②
- The R wave is thus bigger than the S wave in the right precordial leads (i.e. the R:S ratio > 1) ③
- Right axis deviation is often present
- Possible right atrial enlargement and 'strain pattern' in the right precordial leads

Pathophysiology

Increased muscle mass in the right ventricle presents as a large R wave in the right precordial leads and a deep S wave in the left precordial leads. If a strain pattern is present it is due to subendocardial ischaemia in the right ventricle.

Clinical relevance

Right ventricular hypertrophy is usually due to a secondary cause, such as pulmonary, tricuspid or mitral stenosis, or severe lung disease with cor pulmonale.

Management

The mainstay of management is to identify and, if possible, correct the cause. An echocardiogram will identify the majority of valvular lesions, whereas a chest radiograph and pulmonary function tests will detect most respiratory disease.

Clinical insight

Causes of an R:S ratio > 1:
- Posterior myocardial infarction
- Wolff–Parkinson–White syndrome
- Hypertrophic cardiomyopathy
- Early transition
- Normal variant

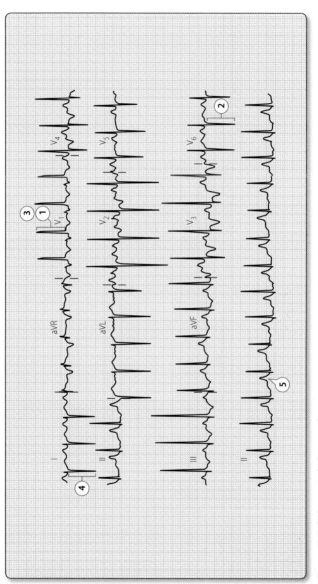

Figure 12.3 Right ventricular hypertrophy.

12.4 Pulmonary embolus (Figure 12.4)

Key features

- Typically an 'S1 Q3 T3' pattern ① ② ③
- Sinus tachycardia is common
- Right bundle branch block morphology may be present
- T wave inversion may be seen in any of the right precordial leads

Pathophysiology

Pulmonary embolism occurs when a venous thrombus, usually in the lower limbs or iliac veins, travels via the inferior vena cava through the right side of the heart and to the pulmonary arteries and lungs. The ECG changes reflect the resulting strain on the right heart.

Clinical relevance

PE classically presents with chest pain, breathlessness and haemoptysis. Small emboli may, however, be asymptomatic, whereas large PEs may be rapidly fatal.

Management

The acute management of pulmonary embolism depends on both its size and the clinical status of the patient. In massive or submassive PE with haemodynamic compromise urgent thrombolysis or embolectomy is required. When the embolism is smaller, anticoagulation with heparin or warfarin is required to prevent further recurrence.

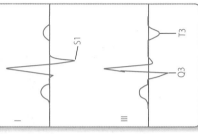

The S1 Q3 T3 pattern

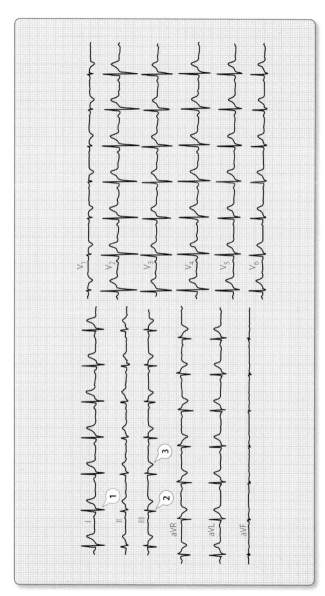

Figure 12.4 Pulmonary embolus.

12.5 Pacemaker (Figure 12.5)

Key features

- The P wave may be normal (it is sensed by the pacemaker) or abnormal (when it is paced) ①
- Pacing spikes may be seen before the abnormal P waves ②
- The QRS complex may be normal (it is sensed by the pacemaker) or abnormal (when it is paced) ③
- Paced QRS complexes are usually broad and have a left-bundle-branch-block-type morphology
- A pacing spike may be seen before the QRS

Pathophysiology

Pacemakers sense normal cardiac activity, and if this is absent will deliver an electrical impulse to cause the atria or ventricles to depolarise and contract. The two most common pacemakers are:

Dual-chamber pacemakers can sense or pace in both the atria and the ventricles, with leads placed in the right atrium and right ventricle. They are commonly used in people with second- or third-degree heart block.

Single-chamber pacemakers sense or pace in the ventricle alone. They are used in AF where neither sensing nor pacing the atrium is useful.

Clinical relevance

Device malfunction is rare, but problems can occur when pacemaker leads become damaged or displaced. Most problems can be identified from the ECG.

Management

Patients are tested every few months, though problems are rare.

Clinical insight

Pacing spikes are not always seen before the P waves or QRS complex, even when pacing occurs. This is due to the way the lead is programmed, and whether electrical impulses travel from the tip of the lead through the chest wall back to the pacemaker box itself (*unipolar pacing*) or they are confined to the tip of the lead (*bipolar pacing*).

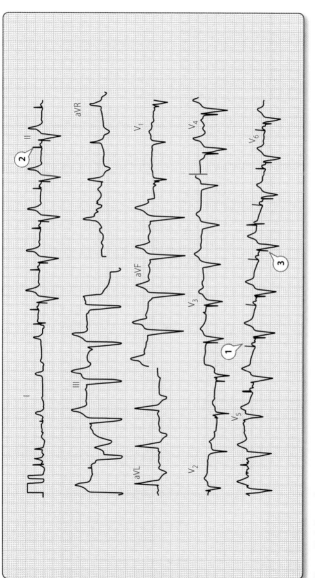

Figure 12.5 Pacemaker.

12.6 Hyperkalaemia (Figure 12.6)

Key features

- Tall, tented T waves ①
- Small or absent P waves ②
- Long PR interval ③
- QRS complex duration prolonged and bizarre ④

Pathophysiology

Hyperkalaemia affects the action potential of cardiac myocytes. Common causes are drugs (particularly ACE inhibitors and spironolactone), renal failure, metabolic acidosis, trauma and Addison's disease.

Clinical relevance

With increasing levels of hyperkalaemia a variety of dangerous rhythms can occur. There is progressive slowing of conduction through the myocardium, leading to bundle branch blocks, atrioventricular block and even ventricular standstill. With advanced hyperkalaemia there is severe conduction delay, giving a sine-wave-like appearance. Ventricular fibrillation may also occur. The P wave becomes progressively smaller, and can indicate sinus arrest or atrial fibrillation.

Management

Hyperkalaemia is a medical emergency. If ECG changes are present, calcium gluconate should be given immediately to stabilise the cardiac myocytes. Drugs and fluids are given to reduce serum potassium levels. The cause for high potassium should be sought and where possible corrected.

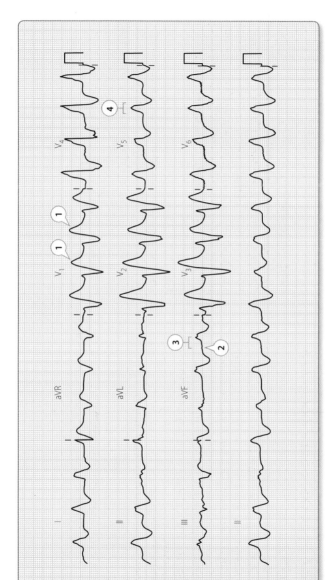

Figure 12.6 Hyperkalaemia.

12.7 Hypokalaemia (Figure 12.7)

Key features

- ST depression ①
- Small amplitude T wave ②
- U wave after the T wave usually in leads V_4–V_6 ③
- Large P wave with PR interval prolongation ④
- Severe hypokalaemia: the QRS complex duration may be prolonged, ST segments may be markedly depressed, and the T wave may be inverted ⑤

Pathophysiology

When serum potassium levels drop to 3.0 mEq/L or below, the cardiac transmembrane gradient is affected and a number of cardiac arrhythmias can occur. These include atrial and ventricular premature beats, sinus bradycardia, atrial tachycardia, AV block, ventricular tachycardia or ventricular fibrillation.

Clinical relevance

In addition to cardiac arrhythmias, hypokalaemia can present as muscle weakness or paralysis, rhabdomyolysis or kidney dysfunction. It is most commonly due to urinary or gastrointestinal losses, but it may be iatrogenic

Management

Potassium replacement is the mainstay of treatment, with the form and rate of replacement depending on the degree of electrolyte disturbance and the presence of cardiac arrhythmias, or any concurrent symptoms. If the magnesium level is low, it must also be replaced.

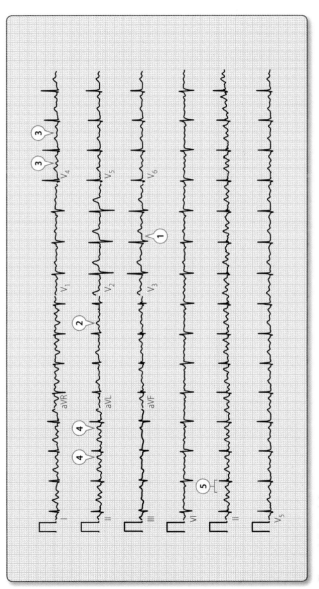

Figure 12.7 Hypokalaemia.

12.8 Hypercalcaemia (Figure 12.8)

Key features

- Short QT interval ①
- Short or absent ST segment ②
- Abnormally shaped T wave with a steep distal segment ③

Pathophysiology

High serum calcium levels shorten the myocardial action potential, resulting in a short QT interval. At very high calcium levels, ventricular or supraventricular arrhythmias can occur, but these are rare. ST segment elevation, mimicking acute myocardial infarction, may also occur.

Clinical relevance

The most common causes of hypercalcaemia are hyperparathyroidism, myeloma and other malignancies. Patients may present with a wide range of symptoms, including polydipsia, polyuria, anorexia, nausea, vomiting and muscle weakness. Aside from the ECG changes described above, cardiac manifestations are rare, but include calcium deposition in the coronary arteries or heart valves, hypertension and cardiomyopathy.

Management

Rehydration with intravenous fluid is the first-line management, with the addition of bisphosphonates later if needed. Wherever possible a cause of the hypercalcaemia should be found and treated. In practice, this means checking parathyroid hormone levels, performing a myeloma screen and investigating for underlying malignancy.

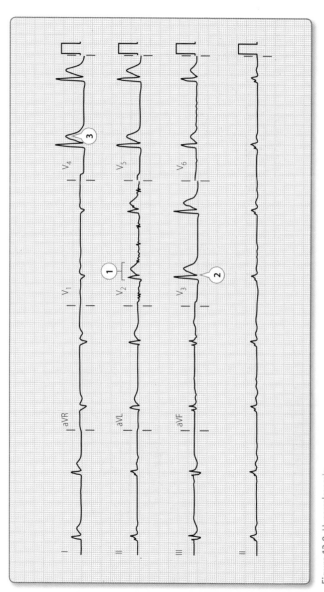

Figure 12.8 Hypercalcaemia.

12.9 Hypocalcaemia (Figure 12.9)

Key features

- Prolonged QT interval with a long ST segment ①
- Small T waves ②

Pathophysiology

Hypocalcaemia prolongs phase 2 of the cardiac action potential and alters myocyte function. The result is a delay in the onset of membrane repolarisation, and this is manifested on the ECG as a long QT interval.

Clinical relevance

Calcium homeostasis relies on balancing absorption from the gut, metabolism of bone and excretion from the kidney. These processes depend on the presence and interaction of a variety of factors, including parathyroid hormone, vitamin D and phosphate. Problems with any stage of this process can alter calcium levels. Symptoms are varied and may be non-specific, but include tetany, confusion, seizures and cardiac arrhythmias.

Management

In the acute setting, calcium can be replaced orally or parenterally. A cause should always be sought, as it may be correctable (e.g. lack of sunlight preventing the formation of vitamin D), and may indicate more serious underlying disease.

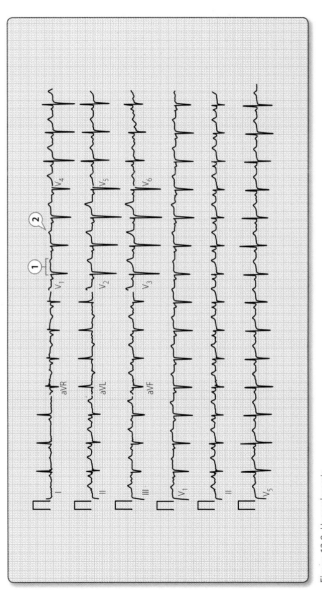

Figure 12.9 Hypocalcaemia.

Index

Note: Entries in bold indicate 12-lead ECGs and their interpretation; page references followed by the letter f indicate illustrations, e.g. 118f.